Contents

Preface

Surgical trainees have always required a comprehensive knowledge of anatomy to complement their development as they progress towards independent practice. While requirements for this knowledge have not changed, exposure at both undergraduate and postgraduate level to teaching in anatomy has diminished as other disciplines compete for space on the curriculum. At the time of postgraduate examinations trainees are, therefore, increasingly finding themselves less equipped to deal with anatomy questions.

As surgical trainees ourselves, when we came to revise anatomy for the MRCS examination we found that, while there were numerous useful reference textbooks available, there was a lack of self-assessment material. We wrote this text in the hope of providing a resource which not only provides relevant material to test a candidate's knowledge base but which also stands alone as a learning text. The questions are of single best answer format and are designed to cover important areas of anatomical knowledge. The answer section provides explanations for each part and highlights learning points.

The development of this project has been greatly aided by the attention and help of Mr Omar Faiz, the editorial advisor for this book. His support and guidance has been invaluable in both improving the format and content of the text, but also in supporting us both in bringing it to publication. We owe him a debt of thanks for his time and effort. We would also like to thank all those at Blackwell who have been involved in the development and publication of this book.

We hope that you find this book useful while preparing for your postgraduate examinations. A lot of candidates find preparing for anatomy questions a daunting prospect and we hope this text will help by focusing your learning and going someway towards building your confidence.

Christopher Wood and Simon Blackburn

1

Upper Limb

QUESTIONS

1.1 Which of the following statements best describes the scapula?
- [ ] **a.** It usually overlies the 2nd to 9th ribs.
- [ ] **b.** The spine continues laterally as the coracoid process.
- [ ] **c.** The suprascapular notch is found on its spine.
- [ ] **d.** It provides attachment for both heads of biceps.
- [ ] **e.** Most fractures involve the body.

1.2 Which statement is the best ending for the following sentence? When considering the humerus, it should be noted that the:
- [ ] **a.** Lesser tubercle has three facets.
- [ ] **b.** Bicipital groove separates the greater and lesser tubercles.
- [ ] **c.** Surgical neck separates the head from the tubercles.
- [ ] **d.** Common extensor origin is the medial epicondyle.
- [ ] **e.** Capitulum articulates with the ulna.

1.3 Which of the following statements regarding the radius and ulna is correct?
- [ ] **a.** Both have a styloid process at the proximal end.
- [ ] **b.** Both articulate with the humerus at the elbow joint.
- [ ] **c.** Both articulate with the carpal bones at the wrist joint.
- [ ] **d.** Direct injury usually produces transverse fractures of both bones in the distal third.
- [ ] **e.** Fracture is most commonly of the Smith's type.

1.4 Which of these statements best describes the carpus?

- ☐ **a.** It is markedly concave from side to side anteriorly.
- ☐ **b.** The most commonly fractured bone is the lunate.
- ☐ **c.** The scaphoid articulates with the 1st metacarpal.
- ☐ **d.** Fracture of the hamate may result in damage to the median nerve.
- ☐ **e.** The pisiform is usually the first bone to begin ossification.

1.5 Which statement most appropriately describes the female breast?

- ☐ **a.** It overlies the 3rd to 8th ribs.
- ☐ **b.** It consists of 2–3 lobules.
- ☐ **c.** It has suspensory ligaments, which tether the dermis to the fascia of the chest wall.
- ☐ **d.** The retro-mammary space lies deep to pectoralis major.
- ☐ **e.** The areolar glands are responsible for lactation.

1.6 Which of these statements best describes the pectoral girdle and shoulder?

- ☐ **a.** The clavicle ossifies in the foetus.
- ☐ **b.** The clavicle most commonly fractures at the junction of the medial and middle third.
- ☐ **c.** The subscapularis bursa is separate from the capsule of the shoulder joint.
- ☐ **d.** The capsule of the shoulder joint communicates with the subacromial bursa.
- ☐ **e.** The short head of biceps lies within the capsule of the shoulder joint.

1.7 Which of the following is true of the rotator cuff?

- ☐ **a.** Teres major is one of its four constituent muscles.
- ☐ **b.** Infraspinatus is innervated by the suprascapular nerve.
- ☐ **c.** Part of its action is to pull the humeral head superiorly.
- ☐ **d.** Subscapularis inserts onto the greater tuberosity of the humerus.
- ☐ **e.** It is deficient anteriorly.

1.8 When considering the axilla, which of the following statements is accurate?

- ☐ **a.** Pectoralis major and minor contribute to the anterior wall.
- ☐ **b.** The long thoracic nerve runs on the posterior wall.
- ☐ **c.** Teres minor forms the lower part of the posterior wall.
- ☐ **d.** The axillary artery lies anterior to the axillary sheath.
- ☐ **e.** The axillary nerve exits through the triangular space.

1.9 Which of these sentences best describes the elbow joint?

- ☐ **a.** The capitulum articulates with the head of the ulna.
- ☐ **b.** The capsule of the joint attaches to the radius.
- ☐ **c.** The annular ligament is attached to the ulna, but not to the radius.
- ☐ **d.** The radial nerve is a posterior relation.
- ☐ **e.** The valgus angle created by the joint is larger in men than in women.

1.10 Which statement correctly describes the cubital fossa?

- ☐ **a.** Its borders are entirely muscular.
- ☐ **b.** A branch of the musculocutaneous nerve is found in its floor.
- ☐ **c.** The median cubital vein traverses its roof.
- ☐ **d.** The median nerve lies lateral to the brachial artery within it.
- ☐ **e.** The radial nerve lies medial to the tendon of biceps within it.

1.11 Which of the following accurately describes the anterior compartment of the forearm?

- ☐ **a.** The median nerve enters the forearm between the two heads of flexor carpi ulnaris.
- ☐ **b.** Palmaris longus is present in approximately 15% of arms.
- ☐ **c.** Flexor digitorum profundus originates from the common flexor origin.
- ☐ **d.** Flexor pollicis longus is characteristically uni-pennate.
- ☐ **e.** The superficial flexor muscles are all innervated by the median nerve.

1.12 Which of the following best describes the forearm?

- ☐ **a.** The median nerve is related anteriorly to flexor digitorum superficialis.
- ☐ **b.** Pronator quadratus lies deep to the long flexor tendons just proximal to the wrist.
- ☐ **c.** The ulnar nerve lies superficial to flexor carpi ulnaris.
- ☐ **d.** Flexor digitorum profundus is partially supplied by the posterior interosseous nerve.
- ☐ **e.** The radial nerve carries motor fibres in the anterior compartment of the forearm.

1.13 Which of the following statements best describes the structures in the posterior compartment of the forearm?

- ☐ **a.** Brachioradialis is innervated by the posterior interosseous nerve.
- ☐ **b.** The common extensor origin is the medial epicondyle of the humerus.
- ☐ **c.** The posterior interosseous nerve pierces supinator.
- ☐ **d.** The extensor retinaculum is attached to the radius and the ulna.
- ☐ **e.** The extensor tendons pass through the extensor retinaculum in the same fascial compartment.

1.14 Which of these statements about the wrist joint is correct?

  ☐ **a.** It is a synovial joint between the ulna and the carpal bones.

  ☐ **b.** The triquetral articulates with the ulna.

  ☐ **c.** The joint line lies at the level of the styloid process of the ulna.

  ☐ **d.** It has palmar, dorsal and collateral ligaments.

  ☐ **e.** The capsule is continuous with the distal radio-ulnar joint.

1.15 Which of the following statements best describes the carpal tunnel?

  ☐ **a.** The flexor retinaculum is attached to the trapezoid.

  ☐ **b.** The tendons of flexor digitorum superficialis lie with the index and little finger tendons anterior to those of the middle and ring fingers.

  ☐ **c.** The median nerve lies directly deep to the tendons of flexor digitorum superficialis.

  ☐ **d.** The palmar cutaneous branch of the median nerve lies superficial to the flexor retinaculum.

  ☐ **e.** The tendon of flexor carpi ulnaris lies within the carpel tunnel.

1.16 The flexor tendons of the forearm run within sheaths in the hand. Which of the following statements best describes these structures?

  ☐ **a.** The fibrous flexor sheaths run from the metacarpal heads to the proximal phalanges.

  ☐ **b.** The annular pullies overlie the interphalangeal joints.

  ☐ **c.** The synovial sheath of the middle finger tendon is continuous with its sheath in the carpal tunnel.

  ☐ **d.** The cruciform pullies overlie the phalanges.

  ☐ **e.** The flexor digitorum profundus tendon pierces the flexor digitorum superficialis tendon.

1.17 Which statement regarding the anatomical snuffbox is correct?

- ☐ **a.** Abductor pollicis longus and extensor pollicis brevis form the ulnar border.
- ☐ **b.** The extensor pollicis longus tendon forms the radial border.
- ☐ **c.** The floor is formed by the scaphoid and trapezoid.
- ☐ **d.** The radial artery runs in the floor.
- ☐ **e.** The origin of the basilic vein is found in its roof.

1.18 Which statement regarding the anatomical spaces of the hand is true?

- ☐ **a.** The thenar space lies lateral to the 3rd metacarpal.
- ☐ **b.** The hypothenar space lies lateral to the 5th metacarpal.
- ☐ **c.** The midpalmar space lies superficial to the palmar aponeurosis.
- ☐ **d.** The pulp spaces lie on the dorsal aspect of the fingers and thumb.
- ☐ **e.** The web spaces lie between adjacent metacarpal bones.

1.19 Which of the following best describes the lumbricals?

- ☐ **a.** The lumbricals arise from the tendons of flexor digitorum superficialis.
- ☐ **b.** There is a lumbrical inserted into the extensor expansion of all five digits.
- ☐ **c.** The median and radial nerves innervate the lumbricals.
- ☐ **d.** The action of the lumbricals is to extend the distal interphalangeal joint.
- ☐ **e.** The action of the lumbricals is to flex the proximal interphalangeal joint.

1.20 The following are statements about the interosseous muscles of the hand. Which is correct?

- ☐ **a.** The palmar interossei abduct the fingers.
- ☐ **b.** There are four palmar interossei.
- ☐ **c.** There are three dorsal interossei.
- ☐ **d.** The dorsal interossei are bipennate.
- ☐ **e.** The palmar interossei are all supplied by the median nerve.

1.21 These statements consider the vasculature and lymphatic drainage of the breast. Which is true?

- ☐ **a.** The main blood supply is derived from branches of the internal mammary artery.
- ☐ **b.** Venous drainage is predominantly to the internal mammary vein.
- ☐ **c.** Lymphatic drainage is divided evenly between the axillary and internal mammary nodes.
- ☐ **d.** The superficial lymphatics of each breast remain separate in healthy people.
- ☐ **e.** All the axillary lymphatics drain through the apical axillary nodes.

1.22 Which of the following statements best describes the subclavian artery?

- ☐ **a.** It is divided into three parts by the scalenus medius muscle.
- ☐ **b.** The second part gives no constant branch.
- ☐ **c.** It is crossed posteriorly by the vagus nerve.
- ☐ **d.** It lies anterior to the subclavian vein.
- ☐ **e.** It is prone to aneurysmal change in the presence of a cervical rib.

1.23 Which of the following statements about the axillary artery is accurate?

☐ **a.** It is divided into three parts by pectoralis major.

☐ **b.** It becomes the brachial artery at the inferior border of teres minor.

☐ **c.** The cords of the brachial plexus are named according to their positions relative to the first part.

☐ **d.** The axillary vein lies medial throughout its course.

☐ **e.** It gives the suprascapular artery as one of its branches.

1.24 The brachial plexus gives rise to the nerve supply of the upper limb. Which of these statements about its branches is correct?

☐ **a.** The terminal branch of the medial cord is the ulnar nerve.

☐ **b.** The terminal branch of the posterior cord is the median nerve.

☐ **c.** The axillary nerve is a branch of the lateral cord.

☐ **d.** The radial nerve arises from the medial cord.

☐ **e.** The long thoracic nerve arises from the roots.

1.25 Which of these statements about the musculocutaneous nerve is correct?

☐ **a.** It is a branch of the medial cord of the brachial plexus.

☐ **b.** It pierces brachialis to enter the anterior compartment of the arm.

☐ **c.** Brachioradialis is innervated by one of its branches.

☐ **d.** The medial cutaneous nerve of the forearm is its terminal branch.

☐ **e.** It contributes to the innervation of the shoulder joint.

1.26 Select the most appropriate ending for the following sentence. The median nerve:

- [ ] **a.** Arises from both the posterior and medial cords of the brachial plexus.
- [ ] **b.** Passes from the medial to the lateral side of the brachial artery in the arm.
- [ ] **c.** Gives no muscular branches in the arm.
- [ ] **d.** Enters the forearm by passing between the two heads of flexor carpi ulnaris.
- [ ] **e.** Supplies all of flexor digitorum profundus.

1.27 Which of these statements best completes the following sentence? The ulnar nerve:

- [ ] **a.** Has the ulnar artery as a medial relation at the wrist.
- [ ] **b.** Passes deep to the flexor retinaculum at the wrist.
- [ ] **c.** Usually innervates the lateral two lumbricals.
- [ ] **d.** Innervates adductor pollicis.
- [ ] **e.** Innervates the skin of the lateral (radial) 1½ digits.

1.28 Which statement considering the relations of nerves to the humerus is the most accurate?

- [ ] **a.** The axillary nerve runs around the anatomical neck.
- [ ] **b.** The median nerve runs in the spiral groove.
- [ ] **c.** Mid-shaft humeral fractures will usually result in complete paralysis of triceps.
- [ ] **d.** The ulnar nerve is related to the lateral epicondyle.
- [ ] **e.** Deltoid may atrophy following shoulder dislocation.

1.29 Consider the dermatomes of the upper limb. Which of the following statements best completes this sentence? The skin over the:

☐ **a.** Clavicle derives its cutaneous innervation from C4.

☐ **b.** Thumb derives its cutaneous innervation from T1.

☐ **c.** Little finger derives its cutaneous innervation from C7.

☐ **d.** Posterior surface of the forearm derives its cutaneous innervation from T1.

☐ **e.** Lateral aspect of the upper limb derives its cutaneous innervation from C8 and T1.

1.30 Which of the following statements ends this sentence correctly? The spinal nerve root mediating the:

☐ **a.** Biceps jerk is C5.

☐ **b.** Supinator jerk is C7.

☐ **c.** Triceps jerk is C6.

☐ **d.** Deltoid reflex is C4.

☐ **e.** Pectoral reflex is C5.

ANSWERS

1.1

d. The long head of biceps takes origin from the supraglenoid tubercle and its tendon runs within the shoulder joint capsule in its own synovial sheath. The short head of biceps arises from the coracoid process via a conjoint tendon with coracobrachialis.

Explanations

a. The scapula overlies the 2nd to 7th ribs on the posterolateral aspect of the thorax. Its medial border runs lateral, and parallel to, the spinous processes of the thoracic vertebrae.

b. The spine continues laterally as the acromion process, which articulates with the clavicle. The spine of the scapula divides the posterior surface into a smaller supraspinous, and larger infraspinous, fossa.

c. The suprascapular notch occurs on the superior border at the junction between its medial 2/3 and lateral 1/3. The superior transverse scapular ligament runs across this notch; the suprascapular artery runs above it and suprascapular nerve runs below.

e. The body is rarely fractured because the majority of the scapular surface is covered by strong muscles and the bone is protected by its association with the thoracic wall. Fractures of the scapula body are therefore associated with high-energy injury, and most fractures involve the subcutaneous, more vulnerable, acromion.

1.2

b. The bicipital, or intertubercular groove separates the tubercles, and contains the long head of biceps and the attachment of latissimus dorsi.

Explanations

a. The lesser tubercle has one facet, which provides attachment for subscapularis. The greater tubercle has three facets, which are the attachment sites of supraspinatus, infraspinatus and teres minor.

c. The anatomical neck is formed by a groove around the head of the humerus, and separates this from the tubercles. The surgical neck lies distal to the tubercles at the proximal end of the humeral shaft, a common site for fractures.

d. The site of the common extensor origin is the anterior aspect of the lateral epicondyle.

e. The distal humerus has two articular surfaces: laterally the capitulum for articulation with the head of the radius and medially the trochlea for articulation with the trochlear notch of the ulna.

1.3

b. The ulna articulates with the trochlea, and the radius with the capitulum.

Explanations

a. Both the radius and ulna have a styloid process at the distal end. The radial styloid is larger and usually projects 1 cm distal to the ulnar styloid.

c. The ulna does not articulate with any carpal bone, but does articulate with the triangular cartilage, the distal end of which forms part of the wrist joint.

d. Fracture of both bones by direct trauma will usually produce transverse fractures at the same level. This would mostly occur in the middle third of the bones as this is the weakest point.

e. A Colles fracture is the commonest form of forearm fracture and classically occurs when falling on the outstretched hand. This results in a radial fracture 2–3 cm proximal to the wrist joint. The distal fragment displaces posteriorly, radially and proximally (impaction), producing a "dinner fork" deformity. A Smith's fracture involves volar displacement of the distal fragment and is less common.

1.4

a. The 8 carpal bones, arranged in 2 rows of 4, form the carpus. The carpus is convex posteriorly and concave anteriorly from side to side. This shape is maintained by the shape of the bones and by the pull of the flexor retinaculum.

Explanations

b. The most commonly fractured bone is the scaphoid. This occurs most commonly as a result of a fall onto the palm, with the hand extended and abducted. The principal blood supply of the scaphoid enters from its distal end. A fracture may therefore interrupt the blood supply to the proximal fragment, leading to avascular necrosis and consequent degenerative change.

c. The scaphoid is one of the four proximal bones of the wrist and articulates with the radius proximally. The trapezium is the carpal bone which articulates with the 1st metacarpal.

d. The deep branch of the ulnar nerve is closely related to the hook of the hamate, and is threatened by a hamate fracture. Decreased grip strength usually ensues.

e. The pisiform bone is a small, pea-shaped, sesamoid bone in the tendon of the flexor carpi ulnaris. Its ossification centre usually does not appear until the age of 9–12 years. It is the last carpal bone to begin ossification.

1.5

c. The dermis is tethered to the breast ducts and the deep fascia overlying pectoralis major by fibrous strands known as the suspensory ligaments of Cooper. As these atrophy and weaken with age the breast becomes more pendulous.

Explanations

a. The base of the adult female breast consistently overlies the 2nd to 6th ribs, from the sternal edge to the midaxillary line. The upper outer quadrant extends towards the axilla as the "axillary tail".

b. The breast consists of 15–20 lobules of glandular tissue, all individually drained by a corresponding lactiferous duct, which empty at the nipple via the lactiferous sinus.

d. The retro-mammary space is located between the posterior capsule of the breast and the fascia over pectoralis major. This space is commonly exploited in the placement of implants.

e. The areolar glands of Montgomery are modified sebaceous glands located beneath the areola and are responsible for lubricating the area. These glands may enlarge or become infected, especially during pregnancy.

1.6

a. The clavicle is the first bone to ossify. It does so in week 5–6 of foetal life.

Explanations

b. The clavicle most commonly fractures at the junction of its middle and lateral third. It is the most commonly fractured long bone in the body.

c. The subscapularis bursa communicates directly with the joint capsule via the gaps between the glenohumeral ligaments. These ligaments reinforce the anterior portion of the joint capsule.

d. The subacromial bursa lies beneath the coracoacromial ligament, and its lower layer is attached to the tendon of supraspinatus. Only if this tendon is torn does the bursa come into communication with the joint. This bursa is commonly injected, both as a therapeutic and diagnostic manoeuvre, when treating supraspinatus tendonitis.

e. The short head of biceps is not directly related to the shoulder. The long head of biceps takes origin from the supraglenoid tubercle of the scapula. It then passes anterior to the head of the humerus within the shoulder joint, enclosed in a tube of synovial membrane.

1.7

b. The suprascapular nerve innervates both supraspinatus and infraspinatus.

Explanations

a. The four muscles which complete the rotator cuff are supraspinatus, infraspinatus, teres minor and subscapularis.

c. The rotator cuff acts to bring the humeral head into contact with the glenoid; thus providing stability, as the shoulder joint has a ball but an incomplete socket. Part of its action is to pull the humeral head inferiorly, opposing the superior pull of deltoid. In a radiograph of a patient with a rotator cuff tear the humeral head is, therefore, seen to lie superiorly.

d. Subscapularis is the only rotator cuff muscle to insert onto the lesser tuberosity. The other three muscles insert onto the greater tuberosity.

e. The cuff is deficient inferiorly. The shoulder joint capsule is also lax inferiorly, because it is attached to the surgical, not the anatomical, neck of the humerus at this point. Dislocation of the humeral head from the glenoid therefore usually occurs inferiorly.

1.8

a. The anterior wall of the axilla is formed by pectoralis major and minor, subclavius and the clavipectoral fascia.

Explanations

b. The long thoracic nerve runs superficial to serratus anterior on the medial wall.

c. The posterior wall consists of subscapularis, teres major and latissimus dorsi.

d. The axillary artery runs within the axillary sheath, together with the cords of the brachial plexus.

e. The axillary nerve runs through the quadrangular space accompanied by the posterior circumflex humeral artery. The quadrangular space is bordered by teres minor, teres major, the long head of triceps and the humerus.

1.9

c. The annular ligament is attached to the radial notch of the ulna and slings around the head and neck of the radius. The radius remains free to rotate within the ligament, allowing supination and pronation.

Explanations

a. The head of the radius articulates with the capitulum. The trochlear notch of the ulna articulates with the trochlea of the humerus.

b. The joint capsule is attached to the humerus at the edge of the capitulum and trochlea posteriorly, and above the radial and coronoid fossae superiorly. Inferiorly it is attached to the trochlear notch of the ulna and the annular ligament, but not the radius itself.

d. The radial nerve is an anterior relation of the joint; it is found at the lateral extremity of the cubital fossa.

e. This is known as the "carrying angle". The larger valgus angle noted in women is required to allow the arm to clear the wider pelvis.

1.10

c. The median cubital vein is a favourite target for venepuncture.

Explanations

a. The borders of the cubital fossa are the pronator teres and brachioradialis muscles and an imaginary line drawn between the medial and lateral epicondyles of the humerus. It is therefore a triangular space.

b. The lateral cutaneous nerve of the forearm is the terminal, superficial branch of the musculocutaneous nerve and lies in the roof of the cubital fossa.

d. The brachial artery lies lateral to the median nerve and medial to the tendon of biceps.

e. The radial nerve lies lateral to the tendon of biceps covered by brachioradialis.

1.11

d. Flexor pollicis longus is one of the deep group of flexor muscles. Its principle origin is from the radius. It is characteristically unipennate, which aids its identification during forearm surgery.

Explanations

a. The median nerve enters the forearm between the two heads of pronator teres. The ulnar nerve enters the forearm by passing between the two heads of flexor carpi ulnaris.

b. Palmaris longus is a vestigial structure, absent in 13% of arms.

c. Flexor digitorum profundus is one of the deep group of flexor muscles and principally takes origin from the ulna.

e. The superficial group of flexor muscles are pronator teres, flexor carpi radialis, palmaris longus, flexor digitorum superficialis and flexor carpi ulnaris. The median nerve innervates all these muscles except flexor carpi ulnaris, which is inner-vated by the ulnar nerve.

1.12

b. Pronator quadratus is attached to the radius and ulnar and lies against the anterior surfaces of these bones.

Explanations

a. The median nerve is found on the deep surface of this muscle, to which it is usually bound with fascia.

c. The nerve lies under flexor carpi ulnaris with the ulnar artery on its lateral side.

d. The anterior interosseous nerve is the branch of the median nerve which supplies the deep flexor muscles: the lateral two tendons of flexor digitorum profundus, prona-tor quadratus and flexor pollicis longus.

e. The radial nerve divides in the cubital fossa. The posterior interosseous nerve carries motor fibres into the extensor compartment of the forearm. The radial nerve continues as a purely sensory nerve to supply an area of skin on the dorsum of the hand. This nerve is often referred to as the superficial branch of the radial nerve.

1.13

c. The posterior interosseous nerve enters the extensor com-partment by passing through supinator.

Explanations

a. The radial nerve gives branches to brachioradialis and extensor carpi radialis longus before crossing the elbow joint, and therefore before the posterior interosseous nerve is given off. In a lesion of the radial nerve below the elbow these muscles are therefore spared.

b. The common flexor origin is from the medial epicondyle of the humerus. The common extensor origin is from the lateral epicondyle.

d. The extensor retinaculum is attached to the radius, the tri-quetral and the pisiform; it is not attached to the ulna.

e. The extensor retinaculum has six fascial compartments. The tendons of the extensor muscles are distributed between them.

1.14

d. The palmar, dorsal and collateral ligaments of the wrist joint represent thickenings of the joint capsule.

Explanations

a. The wrist joint is a synovial joint between the radius, the articular disc and the scaphoid, lunate and triquetral bones.

b. The triquetral articulates with the articular disc of the inferior radioulnar joint.

c. The joint line lies at the level of the styloid process of the radius, which can easily be palpated. This is a useful surface landmark when injecting the wrist joint.

e. The distal radioulnar joint is a synovial joint and its capsule is not continuous with the radiocarpal joint. The two joints are separated from each other by the articular disc.

1.15

d. This fact allows a lesion of the median nerve within the carpal tunnel to be distinguished from a more proximal median nerve lesion, as sensation to the palm will be spared.

Explanations

a. The flexor retinaculum is attached laterally to the scaphoid and trapezium, and medially to the hamate and pisiform.

b. The tendons of flexor digitorum superficialis are arranged within the carpel tunnel with middle and ring finger tendons anterior to those of the little and index fingers. The tendons of flexor digitorum profundus lie in a row, deep to the superficialis tendons.

c. The median nerve is the most superficial structure within the carpal tunnel. It lies deep to flexor digitorum superficialis in the forearm and then passes lateral and superior to it as it passes distally.

e. The tendon of flexor carpi ulnaris, which inserts into the pisiform, is superficial to the carpel tunnel. The tunnel does, however, contain the tendon of flexor carpi radialis.

1.16

e. The flexor digitorum superficialis tendon splits to enclose the profundus tendon as it inserts into the middle phalanx of the finger. The profundus tendon continues to insert into the base of the distal phalanx.

Explanations

a. The fibrous flexor sheaths run from the metacarpal heads to the distal phalanges. They are occupied by the tendons of flexors digitorum superficialis and profundus in the fingers and the tendon of flexor pollicis longus in the thumb.

b. The annular pullies overlie the phalanges and consist of strong transverse sheath fibres.

c. In the index, middle and ring fingers there is a gap between the common flexor sheath in the carpal tunnel and the synovial sheaths of the fingers. The sheaths of the thumb and little finger are continuous with those of the carpal tunnel.

d. The cruciform pullies overlie the interphalangeal joints and consist of loose fibres which are arranged obliquely.

1.17

d. The pulse of the radial artery is palpable in the floor of the snuffbox.

Explanations

a. The radial border of the snuffbox is formed by the tendons of these two muscles.

b. The tendon forms the ulnar border after winding around the dorsal tubercle (of Lister). At this level it gains a blood supply from branches of the anterior interosseous artery. The tendon may undergo necrosis and rupture after a Colles fracture if these blood vessels are disrupted.

c. The floor is formed by the radial styloid, the scaphoid and the trapezium.

e. The origin of the cephalic vein is in the roof. The constant position of the vein at this point makes it a popular target for intravenous cannulation; the so called "Houseman's vein".

1.18

a. The thenar space lies lateral to the lateral septum of the palmar aponeurosis which is attached to the middle metacarpal bone.

Explanations

b. The hypothenar space lies medial to the medial septum of the palmar aponeurosis which is attached to the 5th metacarpal bone.

c. The midpalmar space lies deep to the palmar aponeurosis between its medial and lateral septa.

d. The pulp spaces lie over the palmar surfaces of the tips of the fingers.

e. The web spaces lie between the bases of the proximal phalanges.

1.19

d. By pulling on the extensor expansion the lumbricals extend both the distal and proximal interphalangeal joints.

Explanations

a. The lumbricals, four in number, arise from the radial side of the tendons of flexor digitorum profundus.

b. They are inserted into the extensor expansions of the fingers only. The thumb has no lumbrical.

c. The lumbricals are supplied by the same nerves as their parent tendons: the ulnar two muscles by the ulnar nerve and the radial two muscles by the median nerve.

e. The lumbricals flex the metacarpophalangeal joints, allowing the fingers to be flexed at this joint while remaining straight. The lumbricals are thought to have an important proprioceptive function, regulating finger position.

1.20

d. The dorsal interossei are bipennate and the palmar interossei are unipennate.

Explanations

a. The palmar interossei adduct the fingers towards a plane running down the middle finger. The dorsal interossei abduct the fingers away from the same plane. This can be remembered using "PAD DAB" (Palmar ADduct, Dorsal ABduct).

b. Only three palmar interossei are required. The thumb is adducted by adductor pollicis and the middle finger cannot be adducted towards itself. Therefore, only the index, ring and little fingers require interossei. These muscles arise from their own metacarpals and insert into their respective proximal phalanges and extensor expansions.

c. There are four dorsal interossei. The spaces in between the metacarpals all contain a dorsal interosseous muscle. The middle two are inserted into either side of the middle finger. The outer two are inserted into the ring and index fingers. The thumb and little fingers have their own abductor muscles.

e. All the interosseous muscles are supplied by the ulnar nerve.

1.21

e. There are five main groups of nodes in the axilla. The anterior, posterior, lateral and central groups empty into the apical group. The apical nodes drain into the subclavian lymph trunk.

Explanations

a. The main supply is via the lateral thoracic and thoracoacromial branches of the axillary artery. The internal mammary (internal thoracic) artery supplies a significant part of the medial aspect via perforating branches. The posterior intercostal arteries also make a minor contribution.

b. Venous drainage follows the arterial supply of the breast and is primarily to the axillary vein.

c. Approximately 75% of drainage is to the axillary lymph nodes, primarily to the anterior group. The majority of the remaining drainage, especially of the medial part, is to the internal mammary nodes.

d. The superficial lymphatics have connections with the opposite breast and anterior abdominal wall. If the normal drainage channels become obstructed by malignant disease, metastatic spread may, therefore, occur to the contralateral breast or axillary nodes.

1.22

e. Smaller cervical ribs tend to cause neurological symptoms associated with pressure on the lower trunks of the brachial plexus, but larger cervical ribs may put pressure on the artery, causing aneurysmal change. This may lead to thrombus formation and consequent embolic occlusion of the distal vessels.

Explanations

a. The subclavian artery is divided into three parts by scalenus anterior. The first part lies medial, the second part deep to and the third part lateral to the muscle. The subclavian artery continues as the axillary artery at the lateral border of the first rib.

b. The branches of the subclavian artery are:

First part	Vertebral artery
	Internal thoracic artery
	Thyrocervical trunk
Second part	Costocervical trunk
	Dorsal scapular artery (variable)
Third part	No constant branches

c. It is crossed anteriorly by the vagus nerve. On the right side the recurrent laryngeal branch hooks around the artery at this level before ascending into the neck.

d. The subclavian vein lies anterior to the subclavian artery throughout its course. This important relation must be borne in mind when inserting a subclavian central line.

1.23

d. The axillary vein lies as a medial relation throughout the course of the axillary artery.

Explanations

a. The axillary artery is divided into three parts based on the relation medially, posteriorly and then laterally to pectoralis minor. The first part gives off one, the second two and the third part three branches (see 1.23e).

b. The axillary artery commences as the continuation of the subclavian artery at the lateral border of the first rib, and ends at the inferior border of teres major to become the brachial artery.

c. The cords of the brachial plexus are named according to their relation to the second part of the axillary artery, that is medial, lateral and posterior to it.

e. The suprascapular artery is a branch of the subclavian artery. The branches of the axillary artery are as follows:

First part	Superior thoracic
Second part	Thoracoacromial trunk
	Lateral thoracic
Third part	Subscapular
	Posterior circumflex humeral
	Anterior circumflex humeral

1.24

a. The medial cord also gives the medial cutaneous nerve of the arm, the medial cutaneous nerve of the forearm, the medial pectoral nerve and the medial head of the median nerve.

Explanations

b. The median nerve arises as the union of a branch from the medial and lateral cords of the brachial plexus.

c. The axillary nerve is a branch of the posterior cord. It gives motor fibres to deltoid and teres minor before innervating the skin over the lateral aspect of the shoulder. This nerve innervates an autonomous area over the deltoid (the "regimental badge" area), allowing the axillary nerve to be tested.

d. The radial nerve arises from the posterior cord. The posterior cord also gives off the upper subscapular, thoracodorsal, lower subscapular and axillary nerves.

e. The long thoracic nerve (of Bell) arises from the anterior primary rami of C5, C6 and C7. This nerve innervates serratus anterior. Damage to this nerve, for example when inserting a chest drain, leads to winging of the scapula.

1.25

e. The musculocutaneous nerve gives a branch to the shoulder joint as it crosses it.

Explanations

a. It is the terminal branch of the lateral cord of the brachial plexus. It therefore contains fibres derived from the anterior primary rami of C5, C6 and C7. The other branches of the lateral cord are the lateral pectoral nerve and the lateral head of the median nerve.

b. It pierces coracobrachialis, 5 cm below the conjoint tendon, to enter the anterior compartment of the arm.

c. It innervates the muscles of the anterior compartment: biceps, brachialis and coracobrachialis. Brachioradialis is innervated by the radial nerve.

d. Its terminal branch is the lateral cutaneous nerve of the forearm. The medial cutaneous nerve of the forearm is a branch of the medial cord of the brachial plexus.

1.26

c. The only branch the median nerve gives in the arm is a branch to the elbow joint.

Explanations

a. It arises, by two heads, from the medial and lateral cords of the brachial plexus. The posterior cord gives rise to the radial nerve.

b. The commencement of the nerve is lateral to the artery. It usually passes in front of the brachial artery and descends to lie medial to it at the elbow.

d. It enters the forearm by passing between the two heads of pronator teres. The ulnar nerve passes between the two heads of flexor carpi ulnaris.

e. It innervates all of flexor digitorum superficialis but only the radial two tendons of flexor digitorum profundus. The ulnar two tendons are innervated by the ulnar nerve.

1.27

d. The other small muscles of the thumb are supplied by the median nerve. The ulnar nerve supplies all the muscles of the hypothenar eminence as well as the medial half of flexor digitorum profundus and flexor carpi ulnaris.

Explanations

a. The ulnar and radial arteries lie between their respective nerves at the wrist, such that the ulnar artery lies lateral to the ulnar nerve and the radial artery lies medial to the radial nerve.

b. It enters the hand, with the ulnar artery, by passing through Guyon's canal, which is superficial to the flexor retinaculum. It is, therefore, commonly damaged in lacerations of the wrist and is also liable to compression at this point.

c. The medial two lumbricals are usually innervated by the ulnar nerve. The lateral two are usually supplied by the median nerve.

e. It supplies the skin over the medial (ulnar) 1½ digits.

1.28

e. Deltoid will atrophy as a result of severe damage to the axillary nerve, which may occur following dislocation of the shoulder. The axillary nerve also innervates teres minor and skin over the lateral side of the proximal part of the arm. Sensory loss in this area suggests nerve damage.

Explanations

a. The axillary nerve (C5, C6) winds around the surgical neck of the humerus, accompanying the posterior circumflex humeral vessels. It is prone to damage in humeral neck fractures or dislocation of the shoulder.

b. The radial nerve runs in the spiral groove, where it is accompanied by the profunda brachii artery.

c. Mid-shaft humeral fractures may damage the radial nerve as it runs in the spiral groove. The branches to the lateral and long head of triceps arise before the nerve enters the groove, and thus only the medial head is affected. The characteristic sign of this injury is wrist drop due to paralysis of the posterior compartment of the forearm.

d. The ulnar nerve passes posterior to the medial epicondyle where it is superficial, easily palpable and prone to injury.

1.29

a. The statement is correct.

Explanations

b. The hand derives its cutaneous innervation from C6, C7 and C8, with the thumb being innervated by fibres derived from C6.

c. The skin overlying the little finger derives its cutaneous innervation from C8.

d. The posterior surface of the forearm is innervated by fibres from C6, C7 and C8. The dermatomes are organised in this order from proximal to distal.

e. The lateral aspect of the upper limb is supplied by fibres arising from C5 and C6. The medial aspect of the upper limb is innervated by fibres from C8 and T1.

1.30

a The biceps jerk principally tests the C5 reflex arc, with a contribution from C6.

Explanations

b. The supinator jerk corresponds primarily to the C6 reflex arc, with a contribution from C5.

c. The triceps jerk is principally mediated by C7, with a contribution from C8.

d. This reflex may be of occasional use, and is elicited by placing the examiner's index finger across the tip of the shoulder on the deltoid muscle belly, and tapping the finger. It solely tests the reflex arc of spinal cord segment C5.

e. The pectoral reflex is elicited by placing the examiner's index and middle fingers on the lateral border of pectoralis major and tapping them with a tendon hammer. It tests the reflex arc of C7.

2
Lower Limb

QUESTIONS

2.1 Which of these statements about the femur is *incorrect*?
- [ ] **a.** The intertrochanteric line lies on the anterior aspect of the bone.
- [ ] **b.** The lateral condyle projects more anteriorly than the medial condyle.
- [ ] **c.** Gluteus minimus is attached to the lesser trochanter.
- [ ] **d.** The intertrochanteric crest is the insertion point for the quadratus femoris.
- [ ] **e.** Gluteus maximus attaches to the gluteal tuberosity.

2.2 Which of these statements about the tibia and fibula is correct?
- [ ] **a.** The medial tibial condyle is smaller and more circular than the lateral.
- [ ] **b.** Sartorius, gracilis and semitendinosus insert into the tibia.
- [ ] **c.** Popliteus arises below the soleal line.
- [ ] **d.** The common fibular nerve is subcutaneous at the neck of the fibula.
- [ ] **e.** The fibularis muscles arise from the anterior surface of the fibula.

2.3 Which statement about the arches of the foot is *not* correct?

- [ ] **a.** The medial arch contains the medial cuneiform as one of its bony elements.
- [ ] **b.** The lateral arch contains the lateral two metatarsals as bony elements.
- [ ] **c.** Flexor hallucis longus is important in maintaining the stability of the lateral arch.
- [ ] **d.** Fibularis longus helps to maintain the lateral arch.
- [ ] **e.** Fibularis longus helps to maintain the transverse arch.

2.4 Which of the following best describes the anatomy of the gluteal muscles?

- [ ] **a.** Gluteus maximus is supplied by the superior gluteal artery.
- [ ] **b.** Gluteus maximus inserts into the greater trochanter.
- [ ] **c.** Gluteus medius is a lateral rotator at the hip joint.
- [ ] **d.** They all take origin from the ilium.
- [ ] **e.** Gluteus minimus is innervated by the inferior gluteal nerve.

2.5 Which of the following statements *incorrectly* describes the relations of the hip joint?

- [ ] **a.** Rectus femoris is a superior relation.
- [ ] **b.** Obturator externus is an inferior relation.
- [ ] **c.** The iliotibial tract is a lateral relation.
- [ ] **d.** The femoral vein is an anterior relation.
- [ ] **e.** Pectineus is a lateral relation.

2.6 Consider the fascia and compartments of the thigh, Which statement is correct?

- [ ] **a.** The iliotibial tract lies superficial to the fascia lata.
- [ ] **b.** The iliotibial tract inserts onto the lateral epicondyle of the femur.
- [ ] **c.** The femoral vein passes through the fascia lata.
- [ ] **d.** There are three compartments.
- [ ] **e.** There are three intermuscular septa in the thigh.

2.7 Consider these statements about the anterior compartment of the thigh, Which of them is *not* correct?

- ☐ **a.** All the muscles of the anterior compartment are innervated by the femoral nerve.
- ☐ **b.** Sartorius flexes both the hip and knee joint.
- ☐ **c.** The quadriceps tendon inserts directly onto the tibia.
- ☐ **d.** Quadriceps femoris flexes the hip joint.
- ☐ **e.** Vastus medialis is of importance in preventing lateral dislocation of the patella.

2.8 Which statement best describes the medial compartment of the thigh?

- ☐ **a.** Adductor magnus, longus and brevis insert onto the linea aspera.
- ☐ **b.** All the muscles of the medial compartment are innervated by the obturator nerve.
- ☐ **c.** All the muscles of the medial compartment take origin from the ischium.
- ☐ **d.** The obturator nerve is split into anterior and posterior divisions by adductor longus.
- ☐ **e.** All the muscles of the medial compartment insert onto the femur.

2.9 Which statement best describes the posterior compartment of the thigh?

- ☐ **a.** The common origin for the posterior thigh muscles (hamstrings) is the ischial spine.
- ☐ **b.** Adductor magnus is a muscle of the posterior compartment.
- ☐ **c.** All the hamstring muscles are innervated by the obturator nerve.
- ☐ **d.** Both heads of biceps femoris take origin from the pelvis.
- ☐ **e.** Most of the skin overlying the posterior aspect of the thigh is innervated by the sciatic nerve.

2.10 Consider the femoral sheath and canal, Which of these statements is *not* correct?

- [ ] **a.** The femoral sheath is continuous with the transversalis fascia.
- [ ] **b.** The sheath contains the femoral nerve.
- [ ] **c.** The femoral canal lies medial within the sheath.
- [ ] **d.** The canal is wider in the female.
- [ ] **e.** The canal contains Cloquet's node.

2.11 Which statement correctly describes the femoral triangle?

- [ ] **a.** Its medial boundary is the lateral border of adductor longus.
- [ ] **b.** The floor is formed by the fascia lata.
- [ ] **c.** The femoral vein passes to lie anterior to the femoral artery at the apex.
- [ ] **d.** It contains the short saphenous vein.
- [ ] **e.** It contains the saphenous nerve.

2.12 Which of these statements about the adductor canal is *incorrect*?

- [ ] **a.** It is the communication between the femoral triangle and popliteal fossa.
- [ ] **b.** It is bordered posteriorly by adductor longus and magnus.
- [ ] **c.** It contains the nerve to vastus medialis.
- [ ] **d.** The saphenous nerve exits the canal medially.
- [ ] **e.** The femoral artery exits through a hiatus in adductor longus.

2.13 Which statement does *not* correctly describe the ligaments of the knee joint?

- ☐ **a.** The medial meniscus is larger than the lateral meniscus.
- ☐ **b.** The lateral meniscus is attached to the lateral collateral ligament.
- ☐ **c.** The transverse ligament of the knee attaches to both menisci.
- ☐ **d.** The anterior cruciate ligament prevents hyperextension of the knee.
- ☐ **e.** The posterior cruciate ligament inserts onto the medial femoral condyle.

2.14 Which of the following statements correctly describes the capsule of the knee joint?

- ☐ **a.** It is thickest anteriorly.
- ☐ **b.** The suprapatellar bursa communicates with the knee joint.
- ☐ **c.** Both the cruciate ligaments lie within the synovial cavity.
- ☐ **d.** The infrapatellar fat pad contains the subcutaneous infrapatellar bursa.
- ☐ **e.** The posterior meniscofemoral ligament arises from the medial meniscus.

2.15 Which statement about the popliteal fossa is *not* true?

- ☐ **a.** Is bounded superolaterally by biceps femoris.
- ☐ **b.** Contains the popliteal artery as the deepest structure.
- ☐ **c.** Usually contains the bifurcation of the sciatic nerve.
- ☐ **d.** Contains the long saphenous vein in its roof.
- ☐ **e.** Contains the formation of the sural nerve.

2.16 Which statement correctly describes the anterior compartment of the leg?

☐ **a.** It is separated from the posterior compartment by the anterior intermuscular septum.

☐ **b.** All the muscles of the compartment are innervated by the deep peroneal nerve.

☐ **c.** The anterior tibial artery arises in the anterior compartment.

☐ **d.** It contains extensor digitorum brevis.

☐ **e.** Tibialis anterior assists in eversion of the foot.

2.17 Consider the lateral compartment of the leg. Which statement is correct?

☐ **a.** All the muscles of the lateral compartment are innervated by the superficial peroneal nerve.

☐ **b.** It contains the peroneal artery.

☐ **c.** It contains peroneus longus, brevis and tertius.

☐ **d.** The peroneus longus tendon grooves the lateral malleolus.

☐ **e.** The muscles of the lateral compartment principally invert the foot.

2.18 Which statement regarding the tendons of the muscles of the lateral compartment of the leg is *incorrect*?

☐ **a.** The peroneus longus tendon runs posterior to that of peroneus brevis at the lateral malleolus.

☐ **b.** Both tendons pass under the superior and inferior peroneal retinaculae.

☐ **c.** They share a common synovial sheath as they pass under both retinaculae.

☐ **d.** The tendons are separated by the peroneal trochlea.

☐ **e.** The peroneus longus tendon passes deep to the long plantar ligament.

2.19 Which of the following does *not* correctly describe the posterior compartment of the leg?

- ☐ **a.** The muscles are separated into deep and superficial groups by the posterior intermuscular septum.
- ☐ **b.** All of the muscles are innervated by the tibial nerve.
- ☐ **c.** It contains both the anterior and posterior tibial arteries.
- ☐ **d.** Flexor hallucis longus takes origin from the fibula, lateral to flexor digitorum longus.
- ☐ **e.** Popliteus unlocks the knee by laterally rotating the femur.

2.20 Which statement, regarding the arterial anastomosis around the hip joint is *incorrect*?

- ☐ **a.** The circumflex femoral arteries usually arise from the profunda femoris.
- ☐ **b.** The artery to the head of the femur is a branch of the femoral artery.
- ☐ **c.** The artery to the head of the femur enters with the ligamentum teres.
- ☐ **d.** The hip joint is supplied by retinacular branches.
- ☐ **e.** Avascular necrosis is common in fractures of the femoral neck.

2.21 Which statement best describes the common femoral artery?

- ☐ **a.** Commences at the midpoint of the inguinal ligament.
- ☐ **b.** Gives the profunda femoris branch within the femoral sheath.
- ☐ **c.** Lies between the saphenous nerve and femoral vein at all levels of the thigh.
- ☐ **d.** Lies over pectineus as it passes under the inguinal ligament.
- ☐ **e.** Becomes the popliteal artery as it leaves the femoral triangle.

2.22 Which of the following associations of lower limb movements and root values is *not* correct?

- ☐ **a.** Hip flexion = L3, L4
- ☐ **b.** Knee flexion = L5, S1
- ☐ **c.** Ankle dorsiflexion = L4, L5
- ☐ **d.** Inversion = L4
- ☐ **e.** Eversion = L5, S1

ANSWERS

2.1

c. Gluteus minimus is attached to the antero–lateral surface of the greater trochanter and gluteus medius is attached to its lateral surface. The principal action of these muscles is abduction of the thigh at the hip.

Explanations

a. The intertrochanteric line lies on the anterior aspect of the femur and is the site of attachment of the capsule of the hip joint.

b. The lateral condyle does project more anteriorly than the medial condyle. This prevents lateral displacement of the patella by the oblique pull of the quadriceps. This lateral displacement is also resisted by the oblique insertion of the lower fibres of vastus medialis.

d. Quadratus femoris inserts into the quadrate tubercle, which is an elevation of the intertrochanteric crest. This lies between the greater and lesser trochanters on the posterior aspect of the femur. Quadratus femoris forms the lower limit of the dissection when performing a posterior approach to the hip.

e. Approximately a quarter of gluteus maximus inserts into the gluteal tuberosity, which is found on the posterior aspect of the femur. The remainder of the muscle is inserted into the iliotibial tract.

2.2

b. The tendons of these three muscles form the pes anserinus, which is palpable on the postero-medial aspect of the knee. They all insert into the subcutaneous portion of the tibia, on the antero-medial aspect of the bone, where they may be harvested for use as grafts in anterior crutiate ligament reconstruction.

Explanations

a. The medial condyle is the larger of the two and is oval in shape. The lateral condyle is smaller and more circular.

c. Popliteus arises above the soleal line, from which soleus takes origin. The flexor digitorum muscle attaches to the lateral side of the bone below the soleal line, while tibialis posterior attaches to the medial side.

d. The common fibular nerve (formerly the common peroneal nerve) is subcutaneous at the neck of the fibula and divides into the superficial and deep fibular nerves deep to fibularis longus (formerly peroneus longus). The common fibular nerve is particularly vulnerable to damage at this site.

e. The fibularis muscles arise from the lateral surface of the fibula. The ridges that border the attachment sites of these muscles give rise to the anterior and posterior intermuscular septa that separate the lateral compartment of the leg from the anterior and posterior compartments.

2.3

c. Flexor hallucis longus is important in maintaining the stability of the medial arch. The tendon passes behind the medial malleolus and passes down to the base of the distal phalynx of the great toe. It therefore draws this arch superiorly when contracting.

Explanations

a. The medial arch is formed by the calcaneus, talus, navicular, the three cuneiform bones and the medial three metatarsals.

b. The lateral arch is formed by the calcaneus, cuboid and the lateral two metatarsals.

d. Fibularis longus runs behind the lateral malleolus before crossing the sole of the foot. It grooves the cuboid on its undersurface as it does so. When it contracts it pulls upwards on the cuboid, supporting the lateral arch.

e. The transverse arch is made up of the bases of the five metatarsal bones, the cuboid and cuneiforms. The complete arch is formed by the transverse arches of both feet, which form half an arch each. The fibularis longus tendon helps to maintain this arch by approximating the medial and lateral sides of the foot.

2.4

d. They originate in sequence from the ilium, from superior to inferior.

Explanations

a. Gluteus maximus is supplied by the inferior gluteal artery and innervated by the inferior gluteal nerve. They both emerge inferior to piriformis after passing through the greater sciatic foramen.

b. Gluteus medius and minimus insert into the greater trochanter of the femur. Three quarters of the gluteus maximus fibres insert into the iliotibial tract and the remaining quarter onto the gluteal tuberosity of the femur. It acts to extend and laterally rotate the lower limb at the hip joint as well as to brace the iliotibial tract.

c. Both gluteus medius and minimus are medial rotators, as they pass anteriorly from the ilium to the anterior aspect of the greater trochanter. Their principal action, however, is abduction of the thigh at the hip.

e. Gluteus medius and minimus are innervated by the superior gluteal nerve, and supplied by the superior gluteal artery. This neurovascular bundle emerges superior to piriformis, having emerged through the greater sciatic foramen.

2.5

e. Pectineus forms part of the floor of the femoral triangle and is an anterior relation of the hip joint. It arises from the pectineal line and inserts onto the femoral shaft, just below the lesser trochanter.

Explanations

a. The reflected head of rectus femoris is attached to the ilium just above the acetabulum. The straight head attaches to the anterior inferior iliac spine.

b. Obturator externus is attached to the outer surface of the obturator membrane and passes under the hip joint and neck of the femur to insert into the medial part of the greater trochanter. It is therefore a lateral rotator of the hip.

c. The iliotibial tract blends with the lateral part of the capsule of the hip joint.

d. The femoral vein lies directly over the hip joint anteriorly.
Septic arthritis of the hip may therefore occur secondary to
venepuncture of the femoral vein.

2.6

d. The anterior compartment contains the quadriceps, the
medial compartment the adductor muscles and the posterior
compartment the hamstrings.

Explanations

a. The iliotibial tract is a thickening of the fascia lata on the
lateral side of the thigh. It is the proximal end of this tract
which splits to enclose tensor fasciae latae. Tensor fasciae
latae tightens the iliotibial tract when the knee is fully
extended. This maintains extension without the need for
prolonged contraction of the quadriceps.

b. It inserts into the lateral condyle of the tibia. The iliotibial
tract provides the major insertion for gluteus maximus.

c. The long saphenous vein passes through the fascia lata
at the saphenous opening. The femoral vein lies deep to
it throughout its course. The superficial inguinal lymph
nodes drain into the deep inguinal nodes at the saphenous
opening.

e. There are three compartments but only two intermuscular
septa. The lateral intermuscular septum separates the anterior compartment from the posterior compartment and the
medial intermuscular septum separates the posterior from
the medial compartment. The adductor magnus muscle is
considered to separate the medial and posterior compartments, as it has an adductor and a hamstring portion.

2.7

c. The quadriceps femoris tendon inserts into the superior
aspect of the patella, and continues to include the patella as
a sesamoid bone. From the inferior aspect of the patella, the
patella tendon then runs to insert on the tibial tuberosity.

Explanations

a. These muscles are quadriceps femoris (vastus lateralis, intermedialis, medialis and rectus femoris), iliopsoas and sartorius. The femoral nerve is formed from the posterior divisions of the anterior primary rami of L2–L4.

b. It is the only anterior thigh muscle which flexes both joints. The quadriceps femoris muscle acts to extend the knee.

d. Rectus femoris, one of the four constituent muscles of quadriceps femoris, takes origin from the anterior inferior iliac spine. It bridges the hip joint and acts as a flexor of the hip as well as an extensor of the knee.

e. There is a tendency for lateral dislocation of the patella due to the valgus angle between the femur and tibia, and the direction of pull of the quadriceps. This is resisted by the pull of vastus medialis, which inserts on the medial aspect of the patella.

2.8

a. All three adductor muscles insert onto the linea aspera. The hamstring portion of adductor magnus inserts onto the adductor tubercle above the medial femoral epicondyle.

Explanations

b. Pectineus is a muscle of the medial compartment but is innervated by the femoral nerve. Its action is flexion and adduction of the thigh at the hip.

c. All six muscles of the medial compartment take some origin from the pubic bone. They are the three adductors: pectineus, obturator externus and gracilis.

d. The obturator nerve splits into anterior and posterior divisions which are separated by adductor brevis. The obturator nerve is formed from the anterior divisions of the anterior primary rami of L2–L4.

e. Gracilis inserts onto the upper medial shaft of the tibia, below sartorius.

2.9

b. Adductor magnus has a hamstring portion in the posterior compartment arising from the ischial tuberosity. It also has an adductor portion and is, therefore, part of both the medial and posterior compartments and is dually innervated by the obturator and sciatic nerves.

Explanations

a. The common hamstring origin is the ischial tuberosity. All of the muscles of the posterior compartment have an attachment at this point.

c. The sciatic nerve innervates all the muscles of the posterior compartment of the thigh via its tibial component, with the exception of the short head of biceps which is innervated by its common peroneal component. Its terminal divisions go on to innervate all the muscles of the leg.

d. Biceps femoris has a long head which arises from the ischial tuberosity, and a short head which arises from the distal part of the inferolateral aspect of the femur.

e. The cutaneous innervation of the posterior aspect of the thigh is provided by the posterior femoral cutaneous nerve (S1–S3). This nerve supplies a larger area of skin than of any in the body.

2.10

b. The femoral nerve lies lateral to the femoral sheath. The contents of the sheath from lateral to medial are the femoral artery, femoral vein and the potential space known as the femoral canal.

Explanations

a. The femoral sheath is formed from the transversalis fascia anteriorly and the fascia overlying psoas and iliacus posteriorly.

c. The femoral canal is a potential space which lies medial to the femoral vein. The proximal end of the canal is known as the femoral ring and is bordered anteriorly by the inguinal ligament, laterally by the femoral vein, posteriorly by the pectineal ligament (of Astley Cooper) and pectineus muscle, and medially by the lacunar ligament (Gimbernat's ligament).

d. This is due to the wider female pelvis. Femoral hernias are therefore more common in the female.

e. Cloquet's node is a lymph node that usually occupies the femoral canal and drains the skin of perineum.

2.11

e. The saphenous nerve represents the terminal branch of the femoral nerve, and runs lateral to the femoral artery in the femoral triangle. This nerve reaches as far as the great toe, and is therefore the longest cutaneous nerve in the body.

Explanations

a. The boundaries of the femoral triangle are the inguinal ligament superiorly, the medial border of sartorius laterally and the medial border of adductor longus medially.

b. The fascia lata forms the roof of the femoral triangle. The floor is comprised of iliacus, psoas, pectineus and the remainder of adductor longus.

c. The femoral vein initially lies medial to the femoral artery. As it descends, it lies progressively posterior to the artery and, therefore, lies behind the artery at the apex.

d. The great saphenous vein runs over the roof of the triangle, but then pierces the roof at the saphenous opening. It drains into the femoral vein within the triangle.

2.12

e. The femoral artery exits the canal through the adductor hiatus in adductor magnus to enter the popliteal fossa. The hiatus is a gap between the hamstring and adductor portions of adductor magnus.

Explanations

a. The adductor canal (also known as Hunter's canal or the subsartorial canal) is a fascial tunnel beginning at the apex of the femoral triangle. It is continuous distally with the popliteal fossa.

b. The floor of the canal is formed by adductor longus superiorly and adductor magnus inferiorly. Anteriorly, the canal is bounded by sartorius medially and vastus medialis laterally. The roof is formed by sartorius and the subsartorial fascia.

c. The contents of the canal are the femoral artery and vein, the saphenous nerve and, proximally, the nerve to vastus medialis (a branch of the femoral nerve).

d. The saphenous nerve exits medially at the apex of the canal, piercing the fascia lata between sartorius and gracilis. Here it meets, and descends in close relation to, the great saphenous vein.

2.13

b. The medial meniscus is attached to, and continuous with, the medial (tibial) collateral ligament. The lateral (fibular) collateral ligament is entirely extracapsular and separated from the lateral meniscus by the tendon of the popliteus muscle.

Explanations

a. The menisci are crescent-shaped fibrocartilagenous structures, which are attached to the tibial intercondylar area and the capsule of the knee joint. The medial meniscus is larger and less curved than the lateral.

c. The transverse ligament of the knee attaches to both menisci, and also to the anterior intercondylar area of the tibia.

d. The anterior and posterior cruciate ligaments prevent anterior and posterior displacement of the tibia on the femur, respectively. The anterior cruciate tightens on extension of the knee, with the posterior cruciate tightening to prevent hyperflexion.

e. The cruciate ligaments take their name from their origin on the tibial intercondylar areas. They cross as they pass superiorly to insert onto the condyles of the femur. The anterior passes to the lateral femoral condyle, with the posterior passing to the medial femoral condyle.

2.14

b. The suprapatellar bursa is formed by the superior extension of the synovial membrane of the knee joint, and thus is of use clinically as a site for joint aspiration.

Explanations

a. The capsule is thickest posteriorly where it is reinforced by the oblique popliteal ligament. The oblique popliteal ligament arises as an expansion from the insertion of semimembrinosus.

c. As with the long head of biceps tendon in the shoulder, both cruciate ligaments and the tendon of popliteus are intracapsular but extrasynovial.

d. The infrapatellar fat pad is intracapsular and contains the deep infrapatellar bursa lying immediately superior to the tibial tuberosity. Both the prepatellar and subcutaneous infrapatellar bursae are extracapsular, subcutaneous structures.

e. The posterior meniscofemoral ligament of the knee arises from the lateral meniscus and runs obliquely, posterior to the posterior cruciate ligament, to insert on the medial condyle of the femur.

2.15

d. The popliteal fossa contains the short saphenous vein in its roof. The vein pierces the roof to drain into the popliteal vein having run up the posterior aspect of the calf.

Explanations

a. The popliteal fossa is a diamond-shaped space bounded inferiorly by the two heads of gastrocnemius: superomedially by semimembranosus and semitendinosus, and superolaterally by biceps femoris.

b. The popliteal artery is the deepest structure in the popliteal fossa. The popliteal vein is immediately superficial with the nervous structures superficial to the vein.

c. The sciatic nerve is classically described as dividing into the tibial and common peroneal nerves in the popliteal fossa. It has, however, been observed bifurcating as high as the gluteal region.

e. The sural nerve is a branch of the tibial nerve which is reinforced by the sural communicating branch of the common peroneal nerve. The sural nerve follows the short saphenous vein down the posterior aspect of the calf before passing behind the lateral malleolus to innervate skin on the lateral side of the foot.

LOWER LIMB: ANSWERS

2.16

b. The muscles of the anterior compartment are tibialis anterior, extensor digitorum longus, extensor hallucis longus and peroneus tertius. The deep peroneal nerve, itself being a terminal branch of the common peroneal nerve, innervates them all.

Explanations

a. The anterior compartment of the leg is separated from the lateral compartment by the anterior intermuscular septum. The anterior is separated from the posterior compartment by the tibia, the fibula and the interosseous membrane.

c. The anterior tibial artery arises from the popliteal artery in the posterior compartment. It passes between the two heads of tibialis posterior and then over the interosseous membrane to enter the anterior compartment. It supplies this compartment and then becomes the dorsalis pedis artery.

d. Extensor digitorum brevis arises from the calcaneus and inferior extensor retinaculum. While it shares a blood supply and innervation with the muscles of the anterior compartment, it arises in the foot.

e. Tibialis anterior inserts into the medial cuneiform and first metatarsal bones and, together with tibialis posterior, is a powerful inverter of the foot.

2.17

a. The superficial peroneal nerve is one of the terminal branches of the common peroneal nerve as it passes around the head of the fibula. The superficial peroneal nerve descends along the back of the anterior intermuscular septum and terminates as the medial and intermediate dorsal cutaneous nerves of the foot.

Explanations

b. The peroneal (or fibular) artery is a branch of the posterior tibial artery in the posterior compartment. It arises 2.5 cm below the tendinous arch in soleus, and descends along the medial crest of the fibula between tibialis posterior and flexor hallucis longus. While it gives perforating branches which supply the lateral compartment structures, it remains in the posterior compartment.

c. Peroneus tertius is a muscle of the anterior compartment.

d. The peroneus brevis tendon lies anterior to the peroneus longus tendon throughout, and as such lies in contact with the lateral malleolus which it grooves. The tendon of peroneus longus does not come into contact with the lateral malleolus.

e. They act to evert the foot and are also weak plantarflexors. They have a notable role in plantarflexion if the tibial nerve is damaged. Peroneus longus also contributes to maintaining the arches of the foot.

2.18

c. They have a common sheath as they pass under the superior peroneal retinaculum; however, the sheath divides as the tendons pass above and below the peroneal trochlea under the inferior peroneal retinaculum.

Explanations

a. The tendon of peroneus brevis lies anterior to that of peroneus longus throughout its course, and hence is in contact with the lateral malleolus.

b. The tendons are held down at the lateral malleolus by the superior peroneal retinaculum, and at the peroneal trochlea by the inferior peroneal retinaculum.

d. The peroneal trochlea is found on the lateral surface of the calcaneus and provides an attachment for the upper and lower parts of the inferior peroneal retinaculum. The peroneus brevis tendon passes superior, and that of peroneus longus inferior, to this landmark.

e. The tendon of peroneus longus runs obliquely as the deepest structure of the sole of the foot, to insert into the base of the 1st metatarsal and medial cuneiform bones. It contributes to maintaining both the longitudinal and transverse arches of the foot.

2.19

a. The muscles of the posterior compartment are separated into deep and superficial groups by the transverse intermuscular septum. Both these compartments must be opened during a fasciotomy. The posterior intermuscular septum separates the posterior compartment from the lateral compartment.

Explanations

b. The tibial nerve is a terminal branch of the sciatic nerve and runs through the popliteal compartment into the posterior compartment through a tendinous arch in soleus. It supplies all the muscles of the posterior compartment.

c. The popliteal artery passes with the tibial nerve into the deep posterior compartment through a tendinous arch in soleus. It then divides into anterior and posterior tibial arteries. The anterior tibial passes to the anterior compartment, and the posterior tibial continues in the posterior compartment, where it gives off the peroneal artery.

d. Flexor hallucis longus arises from the fibula, and flexor digitorum longus arises from the tibia. Their tendons cross on the plantar surface of the foot to attach to their respective target digits.

e. Popliteus unlocks the knee by laterally rotating the femur on the fixed tibia. If the tibia is not fixed, popliteus acts to medially rotate the tibia.

2.20

b. The artery to the head of the femur or artery of the ligamentum teres is a branch of the obturator artery.

Explanations

a. The medial and lateral circumflex arteries are usually branches of the profunda femoris artery. They then subdivide to form a rich anastomosis around the hip joint.

c. It runs with the ligamentum teres into the fovea on the head of the femur. It is essential in children when the femoral head is separated from the neck by cartilage, when conditions leading to thrombosis of this artery result in avascular necrosis of the femoral head (Perthe's disease).

d. The main blood supply of the hip joint in adults is by the trochanteric anastomosis formed by the descending branch of the superior gluteal artery, the ascending branches of the circumflex femoral arteries and, usually, a contribution from the inferior gluteal artery. Branches from this anastomosis travel in reflections of the capsule (retinaculae) along the neck of the femur towards the head.

e. The retinacular branches run around the femoral neck, and are commonly damaged following intracapsular fractures in this area. When this occurs and the proximal supply from the artery of the ligamentum teres is insufficient, the femoral head will be at risk of avascular necrosis.

2.21

c. The femoral vein initially lies medial to the artery, and moves to lie posteriorly as they descend. The saphenous nerve is the terminal branch of the femoral nerve and initially lies lateral to the artery, passing anteriorly as it descends.

Explanations

a. The common femoral artery is the continuation of the external iliac artery and commences beneath the inguinal ligament at the mid-inguinal point. This landmark is halfway between the anterior superior iliac spine and the symphysis pubis. The midpoint of the inguinal ligament is the landmark for the deep inguinal ring.

b. This is the main branch of the common femoral artery and arises just inferior to the termination of the femoral sheath (approximately 3.5 cm below the inguinal ligament). The profunda femoris passes posteriorly between pectineus and adductor longus to supply the deep structures, along with the medial and posterior compartments, with arterial blood.

d. It overlies the tendon of psoas. It is separated from pectineus by the femoral vein.

e. At the apex of the femoral triangle the superficial femoral artery enters the adductor canal in which it descends. At the distal end of the adductor canal it becomes the popliteal artery on passing through the adductor hiatus into the popliteal fossa.

2.22

a. Hip flexion is achieved mainly by iliopsoas which is segmentally innervated by L2 and L3. Knee extension is accomplished by quadriceps, which is segmentally innervated by L3 and L4 (femoral nerve).

Explanations

b. Knee flexion is primarily facilitated by the action of the hamstring muscles which are segmentally innervated by L5 and S1 (sciatic nerve). Hip extension has the root value L4 and L5.

c. Ankle dorsiflexion is achieved by muscles of the anterior compartment of the leg, which are innervated by L4 and L5 (deep peroneal nerve). Ankle plantarflexion, achieved by the action of the muscles of the posterior compartment of the leg, corresponds to segmental innervation from levels S1 and S2 (tibial nerve).

d. Inversion is principally due to action of tibialis anterior (deep peroneal nerve) and tibialis posterior (tibial nerve). This corresponds to segmental innervation by the L4 roots.

e. Eversion is achieved primarily by muscles of the lateral compartment of the leg, which are segmentally innervated by L5 and S1 (superficial peroneal nerve).

3

Thorax

QUESTIONS

3.1 Which of the following statements about the surface anatomy of the chest is correct?

☐ **a.** The manubrium overlies the aortic arch at the level of T4–T5.

☐ **b.** The body of the sternum overlies the heart at the level of T5–T8.

☐ **c.** The most prominent vertebral spinous process encountered when palpating the spine is that of C6.

☐ **d.** The manubriosternal joint is at the level of the junction of T3 and T4.

☐ **e.** The xiphisternal joint is at the level of T8.

3.2 Consider the surface markings of the pleura, which of the following is correct?

☐ **a.** The right and left pleura come into contact in the midline at the level of the jugular notch (suprasternal notch).

☐ **b.** The apex of the pleura is approximately level with the clavicle.

☐ **c.** The right pleura passes across the 10th rib in the anterior axillary line.

☐ **d.** The left pleura arches laterally at the level of the 4th costal cartilage.

☐ **e.** The pleura terminates above the level of the 12th rib.

3.3 Which statement about the ribs is accurate?

- [ ] **a.** The head of a typical rib articulates with the transverse costal facet of its own vertebra.
- [ ] **b.** The 8th, 9th and 10th ribs are false ribs.
- [ ] **c.** The 1st rib has the subclavian artery as an inferior relation.
- [ ] **d.** The costotransverse ligaments pass from the transverse process of the vertebra to the head of the rib.
- [ ] **e.** The intercostal neurovascular bundle has the intercostal vein as the most inferior structure.

3.4 Which of the following statements correctly describes the arterial supply of the body wall?

- [ ] **a.** The internal thoracic artery supplies the anterior body wall as far down as the umbilicus.
- [ ] **b.** The first nine anterior intercostal arteries are direct branches of the internal thoracic artery.
- [ ] **c.** The posterior intercostal arteries are all branches of the thoracic aorta.
- [ ] **d.** The lower anterior abdominal wall is supplied by a branch of the internal iliac artery.
- [ ] **e.** The intercostal veins lie directly superior to the intercostal nerves.

3.5 Which statement regarding the internal thoracic artery is correct?

- [ ] **a.** It is a branch of the aorta.
- [ ] **b.** It arises from the brachiocephalic artery on the right side.
- [ ] **c.** It lies between the external and internal intercostal muscles.
- [ ] **d.** It contributes to the blood supply of the breast.
- [ ] **e.** The pericardiophrenic artery is a terminal branch.

3.6 Which of the following statements best describes the lungs?

- [ ] **a.** Both main bronchi enter the roots of their respective lungs at the level of T6.
- [ ] **b.** The left main bronchus gives its upper lobe bronchus before joining the lung.
- [ ] **c.** The blood supply of the lung is derived from the pulmonary arteries.
- [ ] **d.** The left lung has a lingular segment.
- [ ] **e.** Blood from the lungs drains directly into the brachiocephalic trunks.

3.7 Which of the following structures does *not* enter the hilum of the left lung?

- [ ] **a.** The left upper lobe bronchus.
- [ ] **b.** The left pulmonary artery.
- [ ] **c.** The bronchial artery.
- [ ] **d.** Branches of the pulmonary plexus.
- [ ] **e.** Lymphatics which drain into the bronchopulmonary lymph nodes.

3.8 Which of the following statements regarding the divisions of the mediastinum is true?

- [ ] **a.** The superior mediastinum lies above the level of the T3/T4 intervertebral disc.
- [ ] **b.** The inferior mediastinum is conventionally divided into three parts.
- [ ] **c.** The descending thoracic aorta is entirely in the middle mediastinum.
- [ ] **d.** The pericardial sac and its contents form the anterior mediastinum.
- [ ] **e.** The phrenic nerves run in the anterior compartment.

3.9 Which of these statements regarding the superior mediastinum is correct?

- [ ] **a.** The right brachiocephalic vein is shorter than the left.
- [ ] **b.** The vagus nerve enters the thorax posterior to the subclavian artery.
- [ ] **c.** The ligamentum arteriosum usually passes from the left pulmonary artery to the ascending aorta.
- [ ] **d.** The thoracic duct passes across the oesophagus within the superior mediastinum.
- [ ] **e.** The left phrenic nerve passes medial to the aortic arch.

3.10 Which of the following statements regarding the trachea is correct?

- [ ] **a.** It commences at the level of C8.
- [ ] **b.** It is in contact with the left vagus nerve in the thorax.
- [ ] **c.** It has a blood supply from the superior thyroid arteries.
- [ ] **d.** It is lined by mucus secreting cells.
- [ ] **e.** It bifurcates at the level of the T2/T3 intervertebral disc.

3.11 Which of the following statements about the oesophagus is correct?

- [ ] **a.** Is crossed anteriorly by the left main bronchus.
- [ ] **b.** Passes through the diaphragm with the left phrenic nerve.
- [ ] **c.** Has a blood supply from the superior thyroid artery.
- [ ] **d.** Has a venous drainage into the right gastric vein.
- [ ] **e.** Has smooth muscle in the lower 2/3 of its wall.

3.12 Which statement regarding the superior vena cava is correct?

- ☐ **a.** It is formed by the union of the right and left subclavian veins.
- ☐ **b.** The azygos vein drains into its posterior aspect.
- ☐ **c.** It drains blood from all structures superior to the diaphragm.
- ☐ **d.** It forms the posterior boundary of the oblique pericardial sinus.
- ☐ **e.** Has a rudimentary valve at its opening into the right atrium.

3.13 Which of the following statements does *not* correctly describe the pericardium?

- ☐ **a.** The oblique sinus is bounded by the pulmonary veins and the pulmonary arteries.
- ☐ **b.** The transverse sinus lies between the superior vena cava and left atrium posteriorly, and the arch of aorta and pulmonary trunk anteriorly.
- ☐ **c.** It contains the entire ascending aorta.
- ☐ **d.** It is attached to the central tendon of the diaphragm.
- ☐ **e.** The phrenic nerves are directly related to its lateral surface on both sides.

3.14 Which of these statements does *not* correctly describe the phrenic nerve?

- ☐ **a.** It innervates the mediastinal pleura.
- ☐ **b.** It innervates the diaphragm from its superior surface downwards.
- ☐ **c.** It passes anterior to the hilum of the lung on the left.
- ☐ **d.** It lies lateral to the superior vena cava on the right.
- ☐ **e.** It has the subclavian artery on its medial side on the left.

3.15 Consider these statements about the heart, which one is *incorrect*?

☐ **a.** The right lateral border is formed entirely by the right atrium.

☐ **b.** The left atrium is visible when the anterior surface of the heart is viewed.

☐ **c.** The inferior surface is formed by the left and right ventricles, together with the right atrium.

☐ **d.** The base of the heart is directly related to the surface of the diaphragm.

☐ **e.** The pulmonary trunk arises anterior to the aorta.

3.16 Which statement about the right atrium is *incorrect*?

☐ **a.** The crista terminalis separates the smooth walled part from the rough walled part.

☐ **b.** The opening of the inferior vena cava into the right atrium is valveless.

☐ **c.** It contains the embryological remnant of the foramen ovale.

☐ **d.** It receives the coronary sinus.

☐ **e.** The smooth walled part is derived from the sinus venosus of the primitive heart tube.

3.17 Which statement about the left ventricle is *correct*?

☐ **a.** The mitral valve is tricuspid.

☐ **b.** The papillary muscles and chordae tendinae anchor the aortic valve.

☐ **c.** It lies posterior to the right ventricle.

☐ **d.** Its wall has a smooth and a rough portion.

☐ **e.** The aortic valve is bicuspid.

3.18 Which statement about the conducting system of the heart is correct?

- ☐ **a.** The sinoatrial node lies in the crista terminalis, next to the entrance of the inferior vena cava.
- ☐ **b.** The atrioventricular node lies next to the opening of the coronary sinus.
- ☐ **c.** The bundle of His divides in the membranous part of the interventricular septum.
- ☐ **d.** The right bundle branch has anterior and posterior divisions.
- ☐ **e.** The sinoatrial node is supplied by the right coronary artery in 40% of cases.

3.19 Which statement about the valves of the heart is correct?

- ☐ **a.** Both the pulmonary and aortic valves are bicuspid.
- ☐ **b.** The 1st heart sound corresponds to closure of the aortic and pulmonary valves.
- ☐ **c.** Closure of the aortic valve is best heard in the left 2nd intercostal space.
- ☐ **d.** The chorda tendinae tether the atrioventricular valves to pectinate muscle directly.
- ☐ **e.** The chorda tendinae prevent eversion of the atrioventricular valves.

3.20 Which statement about the right coronary artery is *incorrect*?

- ☐ **a.** Supplies the atrioventricular node in 90% of cases.
- ☐ **b.** Usually gives off the posterior interventricular artery.
- ☐ **c.** Contributes to the posterior interventricular artery in a co-dominant circulation.
- ☐ **d.** Anastomoses with the circumflex branch of the left coronary artery.
- ☐ **e.** Arises from the right posterior aortic sinus.

3.21 Which statement regarding the left coronary artery is *incorrect*?

☐ **a.** Is usually shorter than the right coronary artery.

☐ **b.** Has an intermediate branch in 1/3 of cases.

☐ **c.** Supplies the sinoatrial node in 40% of cases.

☐ **d.** Gives off the posterior interventricular artery in a left dominant circulation.

☐ **e.** Passes posterior to the left auricle.

3.22 Which statement *incorrectly* describes the venous drainage of the heart?

☐ **a.** Venae cordis minimae drain into all four chambers.

☐ **b.** The anterior cardiac veins drain into the right atrium.

☐ **c.** The coronary sinus lies in the posterior interventricular groove.

☐ **d.** The middle cardiac vein is a tributary of the coronary sinus.

☐ **e.** The small cardiac vein is a tributary of the coronary sinus.

3.23 Which statement about the primitive aortic arches is correct?

☐ **a.** The first arches persist.

☐ **b.** The second arches become the carotids.

☐ **c.** The third arches disappear.

☐ **d.** The fourth arch links up with the descending aorta on the left side.

☐ **e.** The fifth arches become the pulmonary arteries.

3.24 Which statement regarding the foetal circulation is correct?

- [ ] **a.** The septum secundum lies to the left of the septum primum.
- [ ] **b.** The ductus arteriosus closes at birth.
- [ ] **c.** The foramen ovale is a defect in the septum primum.
- [ ] **d.** The ligamentum teres is the embryological remnant of the right umbilical vein.
- [ ] **e.** The umbilical arteries are derived from branches of the external iliac arteries.

3.25 Which statement concerning the azygos system is *incorrect*?

- [ ] **a.** It comprises veins on either side of the thoracic spine.
- [ ] **b.** The azygos vein passes through the diaphragm with the aorta.
- [ ] **c.** The hemiazygos vein passes through the diaphragm with the aorta.
- [ ] **d.** The anterior intercostal veins are tributaries of the hemiazygos vein.
- [ ] **e.** The hemiazygos and accessory hemiazygos veins drain into the azygos vein.

3.26 Which of the following statements does *not* correctly describe the thoracic duct?

- [ ] **a.** It originates from the cisterna chyli.
- [ ] **b.** It passes through the diaphragm with the aorta.
- [ ] **c.** It drains all the body tissue below the diaphragm.
- [ ] **d.** It usually drains the entire left side of the body.
- [ ] **e.** It empties into the left subclavian artery.

3.27 Which of these statements about the descending aorta is correct?

☐ **a.** The descending aorta forms at the level of T6.

☐ **b.** The aortic hiatus is at the level of T10.

☐ **c.** The aorta usually gives rise to the majority of the posterior intercostal arteries.

☐ **d.** Isolated coarctation usually occurs at the level of the hiatus.

☐ **e.** Gives rise to a pair of subcostal arteries below the diaphragm.

3.28 Which of the following statements regarding the thoracic sympathetic chain is *incorrect*?

☐ **a.** It crosses the neck of the 1st rib.

☐ **b.** It exits the thorax by passing beneath the lateral arcuate ligament.

☐ **c.** It gives off the splanchnic nerves.

☐ **d.** It gives post-ganglionic fibres to the thoracic viscera.

☐ **e.** The first thoracic ganglion may be involved in the formation of the stellate ganglion.

3.29 Which statement correctly describes the left vagus nerve?

☐ **a.** It is the most anterior structure in the carotid sheath.

☐ **b.** It gives a recurrent laryngeal branch which hooks around the left subclavian artery.

☐ **c.** It passes posterior to the aortic arch.

☐ **d.** It passes anterior to the root of the left lung.

☐ **e.** Its fibres pass to the oesophagus to form the oesophageal plexus.

3.30 Which of the following statements best describes the diaphragm?

☐ **a.** It is attached to the xiphoid.

☐ **b.** It is attached to the upper three lumbar vertebrae on the left.

☐ **c.** The oesophagus passes through it at the level of T8.

☐ **d.** The left phrenic nerve pierces the diaphragm with the inferior vena cava.

☐ **e.** A congenital Bochdalek hernia occurs anteriorly.

ANSWERS

3.1

b. The body of the sternum (sometimes referred to as the gladiolus) overlies the heart at this level. This is the anatomical basis of cardiac compressions used in CPR.

Explanations

a. The manubrium overlies the aortic arch at the level of T3 and T4.

c. The most prominent cervical spinous process to be encountered is that of C7 (vertebrae prominens).

d. The manubriosternal joint is at the level of the joint between T4 and T5.

e. This xiphisternal joint lies at the level of T9.

3.2

d. This means that the medial ends of the 4th and 5th intercostal spaces lie directly over pericardium, and a needle passed through these spaces will enter the pericardium without damaging the pleura. With the exception of this arch the surface markings of the left pleura are the same as the right.

Explanations

a. The pleurae come into contact at the level of the sternal angle.

b. The apex of the pleura is approximately 2.5 cm above the clavicle. This renders it liable to damage in central line insertion or in operations on the neck.

c. The pleura crosses the 10th rib in the mid-axillary line. It crosses the mid-clavicular line at the level of the 8th rib and the lateral border of erector spinae at the level of the 12th rib.

e. The pleura reaches the level of the 12th rib posteriorly, which renders it liable to damage in a loin incision.

3.3

b. They are so described because their costal cartilage does not articulate directly with the sternum, but with the costal cartilage of the ribs above. The 11th and 12th ribs are known as floating ribs as they have no costal cartilage.

Explanations

a. The head of the rib articulates with the superior costal facet of its own vertebra.

c. The subclavian artery passes over the 1st rib, posterior to scalenus anterior. The subclavian vein passes anterior to scalenus anterior.

d. The costotransverse ligament passes from the transverse process of the vertebra to the neck of the rib.

e. The intercostal neurovascular bundle runs vein, artery, nerve from superior to inferior and is located in the subcostal groove on the inferior surface of the corresponding rib.

3.4

a. The internal thoracic artery, a branch of the first part of the subclavian artery, runs down the posterior aspect of the sternum and gives the superior epigastric artery and musculophrenic arteries as its terminal branches. The superior epigastric artery runs posterior to rectus abdominis and supplies the body wall as far down as the umbilicus.

Explanations

b. The first six anterior intercostal arteries are direct branches of the internal thoracic arteries. The 7th to 9th anterior intercostal arteries are branches of the musculophrenic artery, one of the terminal branches of the internal thoracic artery.

c. The first two posterior intercostal arteries are branches of the superior intercostal artery, which arises from the costocervical trunk, a branch of the second part of the subclavian artery.

d. The lower abdominal wall is supplied by the inferior epigastric artery, a branch of the external iliac artery, which runs up the posterior aspect of rectus abdominis and anastomoses with the superior epigastric artery at the level of the umbilicus.

e. The intercostal neurovascular bundle is arranged with the vein most superior the artery in the middle and the nerve inferiorly.

3.5

d. The internal thoracic artery has perforating branches which supply the breast. This artery is sometimes referred to as the internal mammary artery.

Explanations

a. The internal thoracic artery is a branch of the subclavian artery. It terminates by dividing into the superior epigastric and musculophrenic arteries.

b. It is a branch of the first part of the subclavian artery on both sides.

c. The internal thoracic artery lies between the internal intercostal and the transversus thoracis muscles. It gives off the anterior intercostal arteries which run in the subcostal groove.

e. It terminates by dividing into the musculophrenic and superior epigastric arteries.

3.6

d. The lingular segment represents the equivalent of the right middle lobe.

Explanations

a. The left main bronchus enters the root of the lung at the level of T6, but on the right side this occurs at the level of T5.

b. The right main bronchus gives its upper lobe bronchus before entering the lung. On the left there are no divisions given before the main bronchus has entered the substance of the lung.

c. The pulmonary arteries deliver mixed venous blood to the lungs for gas exchange. The lung itself is supplied with blood by the bronchial arteries, direct branches from the descending aorta.

e. The right bronchial vein drains into the azygos vein, and the left bronchial vein into the accessory hemiazygos vein.

3.7

a. The left main bronchus divides within the lung after it has passed through the hilum. This is different on the right, where the upper lobe bronchus is given off before the hilum.

Explanations

b. This is correct with two corresponding pulmonary veins draining the left lung and emptying directly into the left atrium.

c. The bronchial artery is a branch of the descending aorta. It supplies the tissue of the lung with oxygenated blood.

d. The pulmonary plexus contains fibres derived from the vagus nerve and the sympathetic trunk. These are afferent sensory fibres from the mucous membrane and efferent fibres to the bronchial smooth muscle.

e. The lung lymphatics drain into the broncho-pulmonary nodes, then pass via the tracheobronchial nodes to the paratracheal and mediastinal nodes. They then drain lymph either directly into the brachiocephalic veins or indirectly via the thoracic and right lymphatic ducts.

3.8

b. The inferior mediastinum extends from the T4/T5 disc to the diaphragm. It is divided for descriptive purposes into the anterior, middle and posterior mediastinum.

Explanations

a. The mediastinum is divided into superior and inferior parts. The superior mediastinum extends from the level of the T4/T5 disc upwards to the root of the neck. The level of the T4/T5 disc corresponds to the surface marking of the sternal angle.

c. The posterior mediastinum contains all the structures below the level of T4/T5 disc which lie posterior to the pericardial sac and its contents. The descending thoracic aorta is the continuation of the arch of the aorta at the T4/T5 disc and runs entirely in the posterior mediastinum.

d. The pericardial sac and its contents form the middle mediastinum. The anterior compartment is the portion of the inferior mediastinum which lies anterior to the pericardial sac, and contains the thymus gland.

e. The phrenic nerves descend from the neck to run on the lateral sides of the pericardial sac, and thus are situated in the middle mediastinum.

3.9

a. The left brachiocephalic vein is longer as it must pass further to drain into the superior vena cava on the right side. The brachiocephalic veins are formed by the union of the subclavian and internal jugular veins, posterior to the sterno-clavicular joint.

Explanations

b. The vagus nerve courses anterior to the subclavian artery at the thoracic inlet.

c. The ligamentum arteriosum usually passes from the left pulmonary artery to the arch of the aorta. It is the embryological remnant of the ductus arteriosus.

d. The thoracic duct initially lies on the right of the midline, posterior to the oesophagus. As it ascends within the thorax it crosses obliquely behind the oesophagus to lie on its left side. This occurs at the level of T5, within the posterior mediastinum.

e. The left phrenic nerve passes lateral to the aortic arch. The right phrenic nerve passes lateral to the superior vena cava.

3.10

d. The trachea is lined by columnar ciliated epithelium, with abundant goblet cells and mucous glands.

Explanations

a. The trachea commences at the lower border of the cricoid cartilage at the level of C6.

b. The left vagus nerve and pleura are separated from the trachea by the thoracic aorta.

c. The blood supply of the trachea is derived from the inferior thyroid arteries and the bronchial arteries.

e. The trachea bifurcates at the level of the T4/T5 intervertebral disc.

3.11
a. This is one of the narrowest parts of the oesophagus as the bronchus tends to narrow the lumen. Foreign body obstruction may, therefore, occur at this point.

Explanations
b. The left gastric vein and the vagal trunks pass through the diaphragm with the oesophagus at the level of T10. The left phrenic nerve pierces the central tendon of the diaphragm as a single structure.

c. There is no contribution from the superior thyroid artery. The inferior thyroid artery supplies the upper third of the oesophagus.

d. Blood from the lower oesophagus drains into the left gastric vein. The anastomosis of this vessel with tributaries of the azygos system is an important porto-systemic anastomosis.

e. The oesophagus has smooth muscle in its lower third only. The rest is formed of striated muscle.

3.12
b. The azygos vein arches over the root of the right lung and empties into the posterior aspect of the superior vena cava.

Explanations
a. The superior vena cava is formed by the union of the right and left brachiocephalic veins. The brachiocephalic veins unite at the level of the inferior border of the 1st right costal cartilage to form the superior vena cava. It ends at the level of the 3rd costal cartilage where it enters the right atrium.

c. It returns blood from all structures superior to the diaphragm except the heart and lungs.

d. It forms the posterior boundary of the transverse pericardial sinus, an important landmark in cardiac surgery.

e. The inferior vena cava has a rudimentary valve at its opening into the right atrium, which is of significance in the foetus as it directs oxygenated blood through the foramen ovale and into the left atrium.

3.13

a. The oblique sinus is a space posterior to the heart and lies between the left atrium and fibrous pericardium. It has the oesophagus posteriorly. It is limited superiorly by a double layer of serous pericardium, separating it from the transverse sinus.

Explanations

b. The transverse sinus is located between these structures as described. The transverse sinus is formed by the folding of the primitive heart tube and allows access to the posterior aspect of the pulmonary trunk and the aorta.

c. The whole of the ascending aorta and entire pulmonary trunk are contained within the fibrous pericardium.

d. The pericardium is securely attached to the central tendon of the diaphragm. It is impossible surgically to separate these two structures.

e. The phrenic nerves pass down the lateral side of the pericardium as described. The phrenic nerves pass anterior to the root of the lung, while the vagus nerves pass posterior to it.

3.14

b. The motor fibres of the phrenic nerve pass through the diaphragm before entering the muscle from below.

Explanations

a. The phrenic nerve is closely related to the mediastinal pleura, which it innervates. It also gives sensory innervation to the fibrous pericardium, the parietal layer of serous pericardium, the central diaphragmatic pleura and diaphragmatic peritoneum.

c. The phrenic nerves pass anterior to the root of the lung on both sides.

d. The right phrenic nerve has venous structures on its medial side throughout its course. It is related to the right brachiocephalic vein, the superior vena cava, the right atrium and the inferior vena cava from above downwards.

e. The left phrenic nerve has arterial structures on its medial side. It is related to the left common carotid and left subclavian arteries, then to the arch of the aorta and left ventricle.

d. The base of the heart is its posterior surface, which is related to the pericardium and posterior mediastinum.

Explanations

a. This is correct.

b. A proportion of all the heart chambers can be seen from an anterior view. The auricle of the left atrium, representing the remnant of the primitive atrium, can be seen above the left ventricle.

c. The inferior surface of the heart is related to the central tendon of the diaphragm and is made up of the left and right ventricles, and the right atrium receiving the inferior vena cava.

e. The pulmonary trunk arises anterior to the aorta, which then arches over it.

3.16

b. There is a rudimentary valve which guards the opening of the inferior vena cava. This valve is of use in foetal life when it directs blood towards the foramen ovale.

Explanations

a. The crista terminalis separates the smooth walled part, derived from the sinus venosus, from the rough walled part, which is derived from the true primitive atrium.

c. It contains the fossa ovalis, the embryological remnant of the foramen ovale, which shunts blood from the right to left atrium in the foetus.

d. The coronary sinus enters the right atrium just next to the opening of the inferior vena cava.

e. The rough walled part of the atrium is derived from the atrial part of the heart tube, the smooth walled part from the sinus venosus.

3.17

c. This is correct; the left ventricle lies posterior to the right.

Explanations

a. The mitral valve is biscuspid, with an anterior and a posterior cusp.

b. These structures anchor the mitral valve.

d. This is a feature of the atria.

e. The aortic valve is tricuspid. The only bicuspid heart valve is the mitral valve.

3.18

b. It lies in the interatrial septum just superior to the entrance of the coronary sinus.

Explanations

a. The sinoatrial node is in the crista terminalis just below the opening of the superior vena cava into the right atrium.

c. The bundle of His divides into left and right bundle branches at the junction of the membranous and muscular parts of the interventricular septum.

d. The left bundle branch has anterior and posterior divisions, the right does not. Bifasicular block is the combination of right bundle branch block and block of one of these two divisions of the left bundle.

e. It is supplied by the right coronary artery in 60% of cases, the left coronary artery in 40% and by both arteries in 3%.

3.19

e. During ventricular contraction the chordae prevent eversion of the valve cusp into the atrium.

Explanations

a. Both have three cusps, as does the right atrioventricular (tricuspid) valve. The left atrioventricular (mitral/bicuspid) valve has only two cusps.

b. The 1st heart sound represents the closure of the atrioventricular valves at the onset of ventricular systole. The 2nd sound corresponds to the closure of the aortic and pulmonary valves as ventricular diastole commences.

c. The closure of the aortic valve is best heard in the right 2nd intercostal space, immediately lateral to the sternum. It is the closure of the pulmonary valve which is heard in the equivalent left position.

d. The chordae tendinae connect the atrioventricular valve cusps to the papillary muscles. Pectinate muscle represents the roughened portion of the wall of the atrium, derived from the embryological primitive atrium.

3.20

e. It arises from the anterior aortic sinus. Nothing arises from the right posterior aortic sinus. The left coronary artery arises from the left posterior aortic sinus. The sinuses lie superior to the respective named cusps of the aortic valve.

Explanations

a. It supplies the atrioventricular node in 90% of cases. Complete heart block is therefore more common following a right than a left coronary artery occlusion.

b. This branch arises as it traverses the posterior surface of the heart. The posterior interventricular artery then descends in the posterior interventricular groove.

c. In a co-dominant circulation the posterior interventricular artery is made up by an equal contribution from the left and right coronary arteries. In a left dominant circulation the posterior interventricular is a branch of the left coronary artery.

d. This occurs in the posterior atrioventricular groove. At the apex there is a further anastomosis between the anterior interventricular (or left anterior descending) branch of the left coronary artery and the posterior interventricular and marginal branches of the right coronary.

3.21

e. The left coronary artery passes forward from its origin at the left posterior aortic sinus, behind the pulmonary trunk and anterior to the left auricle.

Explanations

a. The left coronary artery is usually 1–4 cm in length and terminates by dividing into the anterior interventricular (left anterior descending) and circumflex coronary arteries.

b. This branch passes between the left anterior descending and the circumflex coronary arteries.

c. The sinoatrial node is supplied by the right coronary artery in 60% of cases and the circumflex branch of the left coronary artery in 40% of cases.

d. In a left dominant circulation the circumflex coronary artery is longer, and gives off the posterior interventricular artery before anastomosing with the right coronary artery.

3.22

c. It lies in the posterior atrioventricular groove and accompanies the circumflex branch of the left coronary artery. The posterior interventricular groove is occupied by the posterior interventricular coronary artery.

Explanations

a. The venae cordis minimae draining into the left atrium and left ventricle represent a physiological shunt as blood passes back to the systemic circulation without passing to the lungs.

b. The anterior cardiac veins drain the anterior surface of the heart and end by passing into the right atrium.

d. The great, middle and small cardiac veins are all tributaries of the coronary sinus.

e. This is correct.

3.23

d. The fourth arch becomes the arch of the aorta on the left side. On the right side it becomes the subclavian artery.

Explanations

a. The first arch disappears early.

b. The second arch disappears early.

c. The third arch becomes the carotids.

e. The fifth arch disappears. The sixth arch becomes the right and left pulmonary arteries. On the left the connection to the dorsal aorta persists, forming the ductus arteriosus.

3.24

b. Functional closure is achieved at birth by active muscular contraction.

Explanations

a. The septum secundum lies to the right of the septum primum. Together these structures form the atrial septum.

c. The defect in the septum primum is the ostium secundum, the defect in the septum secundum is the foramen ovale.

d. It is the embryological remnant of the left umbilical vein.

e. The umbilical arteries are derived from the superior vesical branches of the internal iliac arteries.

3.25

d. These veins are tributaries of the internal thoracic vein. The posterior intercostal veins are tributaries of the azygos, hemiazygos and accessory hemiazygos veins.

Explanations

a. The azygos vein lies on the right of the thoracic spine, the hemiazygos and accessory hemiazygos veins lie on the left.

b. The aorta passes through the diaphragm with the azygos vein, hemiazygos vein and the thoracic duct at the level of T12.

c. This is correct.

e. The hemiazygos and accessory hemiazygos veins cross the midline to drain into the azygos vein. The azygos vein then arches anteriorly to empty into the posterior aspect of the superior vena cava.

3.26

e. It drains into the junction between the left subclavian vein and left internal jugular vein. The right lymphatic duct, draining the right side of the head, upper limb and right upper thorax, empties at an equivalent point on the right side.

Explanations

a. It originates from the confluence of sinuses, or cisterna chyli, which lies lateral to the aorta at the level of T12 on the right side.

b. It passes posterior to the right crus of the diaphragm at the level of T12, to lie between the azygos vein on its right side and thoracic aorta on its left. It moves to the left as it ascends, crossing the midline posterior to the oesophagus at the level of T5.

c. The lymph from the lower limbs and abdomen all drains into the cisterna chyli, which empties into the thoracic duct.

d. The left jugular, subclavian and mediastinal lymph trunks drain the left head, upper limb and thorax. These usually empty into the thoracic duct, but occasionally drain separately into veins in the neck. On the right side similar trunks drain into the right lymphatic duct.

3.27
c. There are usually nine pairs of posterior intercostal arteries arising from the descending thoracic aorta, which pass into the 3rd to 11th intercostal spaces. The first two are derived from the superior intercostal branch of the costocervical trunk.

Explanations
a. The descending aorta forms at the level of T4 and is the continuation of the arch of the aorta.

b. The thoracic aorta passes through the aortic hiatus in the diaphragm to continue as the abdominal aorta anterior to the inferior border of T12. It is accompanied on its right side by the thoracic duct and azygos vein.

d. The commonest site for a coarctation is near the insertion of the ductus arteriosus. If it develops inferior to this a good collateral circulation usually develops via the inter-costal and internal thoracic arteries. The collateral vessels may become so enlarged that they may erode the adjacent ribs, which can be visualised as notching on a chest radiograph.

e. This pair arises in series with the intercostal arteries above the diaphragm and runs inferior to the 12th rib.

3.28
b. It passes under the medial arcuate ligament. The subcostal neurovascular bundle passes under the lateral arcuate ligament.

Explanations
a. The sympathetic chain crosses the neck of the 1st rib, the heads of the 2nd to 10th ribs and the bodies of T11 and T12.

c. The splanchnic nerves (formed from T5 to T12) contain pre-ganglionic fibres which pass to the coeliac and renal ganglia. Postganglionic fibres then pass to the abdominal organs.

d. These fibres arise from T1 to T5.

e. It does so by combining with the inferior cervical ganglion. The stellate ganglion is found in front of the neck of the 1st rib and is a useful landmark in thoracoscopic sympathectomy. Interruption of the cervical sympathetic pathway results in a Horner's syndrome.

3.29

e. The vagi break up on the oesophagus at the level of the oesophageal hiatus to form a plexus, from which are derived the anterior and posterior vagal trunks.

Explanations

a. It is the most posterior structure in the carotid sheath, and thus emerges in the superior mediastinum from behind the left common carotid artery and left internal jugular vein.

b. The left recurrent laryngeal nerve hooks around the aortic arch and the ligamentum arteriosum, which represents the remnant of the foetal ductus arteriosus and connects the left pulmonary trunk to the aortic arch.

c. It passes anterior to the aortic arch as it descends, where it gives off its recurrent laryngeal branch.

d. After running anteriorly over the aortic arch, it passes posterior to the root of the left lung on its path into the posterior mediastinum.

3.30

a. The diaphragm is attached to the xiphoid via two slips.

Explanations

b. The right crus attaches to the upper three lumbar vertebrae and the left crus attaches to the upper two lumbar vertebrae. The splanchnic nerves enter the abdomen by piercing the crura.

c. It passes through the diaphragm at the level of T10 and is accompanied by the vagal trunks. The inferior vena cava passes through the central tendon at the level of T8.

d. The right phrenic nerve passes through the diaphragm with the inferior vena cava. The left pierces the central tendon independently.

e. The diaphragm is formed from the septum transversum (forming the central tendon), pleuroperitoneal membranes, a contribution from the body wall and the dorsal oesophageal mesentery. Failure of the development of the pleuroperitoneal membrane leads to the commoner Bochdalek hernia. This occurs posteriorly, more commonly on the left side. A Morgagni hernia occurs at the junction of the costal and xiphoid origins.

4

Abdomen

QUESTIONS

4.1 Which statement best describes the planes of the abdomen?

- ☐ **a.** The transpyloric plane lies halfway between the xiphoid and the symphysis pubis.
- ☐ **b.** The transpyloric plane passes through the hilar of the kidneys.
- ☐ **c.** The subcostal plane is at the level of the body of L2.
- ☐ **d.** The iliac crests lie at the level of L5.
- ☐ **e.** The umbilicus usually lies at the level of the L4/L5 disc.

4.2 Which statement about the regions of the abdomen is correct?

- ☐ **a.** The epigastrium lies medial to the mid-clavicular line and above the transpyloric plane.
- ☐ **b.** The suprapubic region lies between the mid-clavicular lines, the transpyloric plane and the intertubercular line.
- ☐ **c.** The iliac fossa lies lateral to the mid-clavicular line and above the intertubercular line.
- ☐ **d.** The hypochondrium lies below the transpyloric plane and medial to the mid-clavicular line.
- ☐ **e.** The mid-clavicular line crosses the midpoint of the inguinal ligament.

4.3 Which statement correctly describes the abdominal wall?

☐ **a.** The superficial fascia of the abdominal wall contains Camper's fascia.

☐ **b.** The deep fascia of the abdominal wall is known as Scarpa's fascia.

☐ **c.** Scarpa's fascia adheres to the superficial fascia of the thigh.

☐ **d.** The umbilicus receives sensory fibres from T8.

☐ **e.** The groin is innervated by T12.

4.4 Which statement about the rectus abdominis is correct?

☐ **a.** It has the transversalis fascia posteriorly throughout its length.

☐ **b.** It has three tendinous intersections which are visible posteriorly.

☐ **c.** It has the aponeuroses of the three oblique abdominal muscles anterior to it below the arcuate line.

☐ **d.** The lower free border of the anterior rectus sheath is called the arcuate line.

☐ **e.** The linea alba is a highly vascular structure.

4.5 Which statement about the oblique abdominal muscles is *incorrect*?

☐ **a.** The fibres of external oblique pass antero-inferiorly.

☐ **b.** The lower fibres of internal oblique form the inguinal ligament.

☐ **c.** The external oblique arises from the lower eight ribs.

☐ **d.** Internal oblique arises from the lumbar fascia.

☐ **e.** The internal oblique has a free lower border.

4.6 Which statement best completes this sentence? The inguinal canal:

☐ **a.** Has a deep ring, which is a defect in the transversus abdominis muscle.

☐ **b.** Is bounded posteriorly by the inguinal ligament.

☐ **c.** Has the internal oblique as part of its posterior wall throughout.

☐ **d.** Has the conjoint tendon superiorly.

☐ **e.** Transmits the ilioinguinal nerve, which enters the canal through the deep ring.

4.7 Which of the following statements about the peritoneum is correct?

☐ **a.** The median umbilical fold contains the obliterated remnant of the umbilical artery.

☐ **b.** The greater omentum consists of four layers of peritoneum.

☐ **c.** The gastrosplenic ligament contains the splenic vessels.

☐ **d.** The lienorenal ligament contains the short gastric vessels.

☐ **e.** The lesser omentum connects the liver to the transverse colon.

4.8 Which statement about the lesser sac is *not* correct?

☐ **a.** It is connected to the greater sac via the epiploic foramen.

☐ **b.** The stomach is related anteriorly.

☐ **c.** The pancreas is a posterior relation.

☐ **d.** The greater omentum is an anterior relation.

☐ **e.** The right border is formed by the lienorenal and gastrosplenic ligaments.

4.9 Which statement about the borders of the epiploic foramen is correct?

☐ **a.** The second part of the duodenum forms the inferior border.

☐ **b.** The quadrate process of the liver forms the superior border.

☐ **c.** The hepatic vein forms the posterior border.

☐ **d.** The free edge of the greater omentum forms the anterior border.

☐ **e.** The common bile duct is contained within the anterior border.

4.10 Which of the following statements regarding peritoneal compartments is correct?

☐ **a.** The infracolic compartment lies below the lesser omentum.

☐ **b.** The right and left subphrenic spaces are separated by the coronary ligament.

☐ **c.** The right subhepatic space lies between the right lobe of the liver and the right kidney.

☐ **d.** The left subhepatic space is also known as the hepatorenal pouch.

☐ **e.** The right paracolic gutter lies medial to the colon.

4.11 Which of these statements about the coeliac trunk is *not* correct?

☐ **a.** It supplies the foregut and its derivatives.

☐ **b.** It leaves the aorta at the level of L1.

☐ **c.** It gives a left gastric branch that supplies the oesophagus.

☐ **d.** It gives a splenic branch.

☐ **e.** It gives rise to the gastroduodenal artery via its hepatic branch.

4.12 Which statement best describes the blood supply of the stomach?

- ☐ **a.** It is derived entirely from the superior mesenteric artery.
- ☐ **b.** The gastroepiploic arteries supply the lesser curvature.
- ☐ **c.** The right gastric artery is a direct branch of the coeliac axis.
- ☐ **d.** The left gastroepiploic artery arises directly from the coeliac trunk.
- ☐ **e.** The short gastric arteries arise from the splenic artery.

4.13 Which statement best describes the venous drainage of the alimentary tract?

- ☐ **a.** All blood drains into the portal system.
- ☐ **b.** The portal vein is formed from the union of the inferior mesenteric and splenic veins.
- ☐ **c.** The superior mesenteric vein crosses the uncinate process of the pancreas.
- ☐ **d.** The inferior mesenteric vein passes behind the left renal vein.
- ☐ **e.** The prepyloric vein is variable in position.

4.14 Which statement best completes this sentence? The superior mesenteric artery:

- ☐ **a.** Supplies the gut from the pylorus to the terminal ileum.
- ☐ **b.** Arises from the aorta at the level of L1.
- ☐ **c.** Runs in front of the body of the pancreas.
- ☐ **d.** Crosses the second part of the duodenum.
- ☐ **e.** Supplies the appendix via its right colic branch.

4.15 Which statement best describes the inferior mesenteric artery?

☐ **a.** It arises from the aorta at the level of the transpyloric plane.

☐ **b.** It supplies the mucus membrane of the gut as far as the mid-rectum.

☐ **c.** It gives off a left colic branch.

☐ **d.** It crosses the pelvic brim at the point of bifurcation of the right common iliac vessels.

☐ **e.** It anastomoses with the superior mesenteric artery via its sigmoid branch.

4.16 Which statement best describes the lymphatics of the gastrointestinal tract?

☐ **a.** They generally follow routes which are distinct from those taken by the venous drainage of the bowel.

☐ **b.** Peyer's patches are found on the mesenteric surface of the large bowel.

☐ **c.** Lymphoid follicles become less numerous in the distal part of the gut.

☐ **d.** Preaortic nodes lie at the origins of major blood vessels.

☐ **e.** Lymph from the alimentary tract eventually passes into the portal system of veins.

4.17 Which statement best describes the stomach?

☐ **a.** Lymph from the superior 2/3 of the stomach drains into the suprapancreatic nodes.

☐ **b.** All lymph from the stomach drains through the coeliac nodes.

☐ **c.** The gastric branches of the vagi are given of in the greater curve.

☐ **d.** The lower oesophageal sphinchter is supplied by the nerves of Latarjet.

☐ **e.** The antral part of the stomach secretes an acid solution.

4.18 Which of the following statements about the duodenum is *incorrect*?

☐ **a.** The second part overlies the right kidney.

☐ **b.** The transverse mesocolon attaches over the second part.

☐ **c.** The ampulla of Vater lies in the third part.

☐ **d.** The inferior vena cava and aorta lie directly behind the third part.

☐ **e.** The gall bladder overlies the first part.

4.19 Which statement regarding the jejunum and ileum is *incorrect*?

☐ **a.** The ileum has thicker walls than the jejunum.

☐ **b.** The proximal small intestine is of greater diameter than the distal.

☐ **c.** The mesentery of the small intestine is thicker distally.

☐ **d.** The jejunum lies mainly in the umbilical region.

☐ **e.** The mesenteric vessels form more numerous arcades in the ileum.

4.20 Which of these statements regarding Meckel's diverticulum is correct?

☐ **a.** It is found in about 4% of the population.

☐ **b.** Is always found on the antimesenteric border of the ileum.

☐ **c.** Is usually about 2 cm in length.

☐ **d.** Is usually located about 20 cm from the ileocaecal junction.

☐ **e.** Is usually attached to the umbilicus.

4.21 Which statement about the appendix is *incorrect*?
- [ ] **a.** The taenia coli converge on the base of the appendix.
- [ ] **b.** The mesoappendix contains the appendicular vessels in its free edge.
- [ ] **c.** The ileocaecal fold connects the appendix to the ileum.
- [ ] **d.** The appendix always lies behind the ileum.
- [ ] **e.** The appendix opens into the posteromedial part of the caecum.

4.22 Which of the following statements best describes the colon?
- [ ] **a.** The majority is derived from the primitive hindgut.
- [ ] **b.** It is usually invested with peritoneum on all sides.
- [ ] **c.** The hepatic flexure is related directly to the liver and right kidney.
- [ ] **d.** The ascending and descending colon are always retroperitoneal.
- [ ] **e.** The appendices epiploicae are composed of lymphoid tissue.

4.23 Which statement most correctly describes the large bowel?
- [ ] **a.** The taenia coli are longer than the colon.
- [ ] **b.** The descending colon is the longest part.
- [ ] **c.** The sigmoid colon has a mesentery.
- [ ] **d.** The parasympathetic supply is entirely derived from the vagus nerve.
- [ ] **e.** The marginal artery lies within the bowel wall.

4.24 Which statement about the liver is correct?

- [ ] **a.** The gall bladder lies directly anterior to the fissure for the ligamentum venosum.
- [ ] **b.** The ligamentum teres contains the falciform ligament.
- [ ] **c.** The caudate lobe lies anterior to the quadrate lobe.
- [ ] **d.** The liver is closely related to the abdominal oesophagus.
- [ ] **e.** The functional lobes of the liver are demarcated by a line drawn between the attachment of the falciform ligament and the fissure for the ligamentum venosum.

4.25 Which statement best completes this sentence? The porta hepatis contains:

- [ ] **a.** The hepatic artery on the left side.
- [ ] **b.** The common hepatic duct anteriorly.
- [ ] **c.** The portal vein anteriorly.
- [ ] **d.** Parasympathetic fibres from the vagus.
- [ ] **e.** Sympathetic fibres from the hypogastric plexus.

4.26 When considering porto-systemic anastomosis, which of the following statements is correct?

- [ ] **a.** The portal vein is formed by the union of the superior and inferior mesenteric veins.
- [ ] **b.** There is an anastomosis between the middle and inferior rectal veins.
- [ ] **c.** There is an anastomosis between the azygos system and right gastric veins.
- [ ] **d.** There is a direct anastomosis between the paraumbilical and common iliac veins.
- [ ] **e.** There is an anastomosis between the colic and retroperitoneal veins.

4.27 Which statement concerning the peritoneal reflections on the liver is *not* correct?

☐ **a.** The bare area lies between the left and right triangular ligaments.

☐ **b.** The coronary ligament is continuous with the falciform ligament.

☐ **c.** The inferior vena cava forms a border of the bare area.

☐ **d.** The lesser omentum is reflected around the structures of the porta hepatis.

☐ **e.** The bare area is in contact with the right suprarenal gland.

4.28 Which of the following statements about the biliary system is correct?

☐ **a.** The pancreatic duct drains into the hepatic duct.

☐ **b.** The common hepatic duct is formed by the union of the common bile and cystic ducts.

☐ **c.** Callot's triangle is formed by the hepatic duct, cystic duct and the cystic artery.

☐ **d.** The common bile duct runs behind the first part of the duodenum.

☐ **e.** The common bile duct runs between the head of the pancreas and the third part of the duodenum.

4.29 Which statement concerning the relations of the kidneys is correct?

☐ **a.** The diaphragm is directly related to the superior pole of both kidneys.

☐ **b.** The left kidney is related to the duodenum.

☐ **c.** The kidneys are posteriorly related to quadratus lumborum.

☐ **d.** The pancreas is related to the left kidney above the stomach.

☐ **e.** The right kidney is related to the descending colon.

4.30 Which statement about the fascia of the kidney is true?

- [ ] **a.** The suprarenals lie in the same fascial compartment as the kidneys.
- [ ] **b.** The renal fascia is continuous with fascia over the inferior vena cava and aorta.
- [ ] **c.** The perinephric fat lies outside the renal fascia.
- [ ] **d.** The lienorenal ligament is attached to the right kidney.
- [ ] **e.** The perinephric fat lies deep to the true capsule of the kidney.

4.31 Which of these statements about the pancreas is *not* correct?

- [ ] **a.** The neck lies in the subcostal plane.
- [ ] **b.** It is supplied by the splenic artery.
- [ ] **c.** The uncinate process drains via the accessory pancreatic duct.
- [ ] **d.** It is related to the second part of the duodenum.
- [ ] **e.** Develops from two buds which arise from the primitive foregut.

4.32 Which of the following does *not* correctly describe the spleen?

- [ ] **a.** Has a notched superior border.
- [ ] **b.** Lies under the 9th to 11th ribs.
- [ ] **c.** Is related directly to the left kidney and the stomach.
- [ ] **d.** Is completely invested in peritoneum.
- [ ] **e.** The tail of the pancreas is related to the hilum.

4.33 Which statement best describes psoas major?

- [ ] **a.** The femoral nerve emerges medial to it.
- [ ] **b.** The obturator nerve pierces the muscle.
- [ ] **c.** The genitofemoral nerve emerges lateral to it.
- [ ] **d.** It is attached distally to the intertrochanteric line.
- [ ] **e.** The medial arcuate ligament is a condensation of its fascia.

4.34 Which statement correctly completes the following sentence? The abdominal aorta:

☐ **a.** Has four lumbar branches.

☐ **b.** Is crossed by the body of the pancreas between the origins of the superior mesenteric artery and inferior mesenteric artery.

☐ **c.** Has the subcostal artery as its first branch.

☐ **d.** Ends at the level of the L5/S1 disc.

☐ **e.** Gives three direct branches to the suprarenals.

4.35 Which statement correctly describes the inferior vena cava?

☐ **a.** It commences at the level of L3.

☐ **b.** It has gastrointestinal tributaries which correspond to the equivalent branches of the aorta.

☐ **c.** The second lumbar vein is a tributary.

☐ **d.** The subcostal vein is a tributary.

☐ **e.** The hepatic veins are tributaries.

4.36 Which statement about the lumbar plexus is *incorrect*?

☐ **a.** It is formed by the anterior primary rami of L1–L4.

☐ **b.** The ilioinguinal and iliohypogastric nerves are both derived from L3.

☐ **c.** The femoral and obturator nerves are both derived from the anterior primary rami of L2–L4.

☐ **d.** A branch of the genitofemoral nerve traverses the inguinal canal.

☐ **e.** It is connected to the sacral plexus by the lumbosacral trunk.

4.37 Which statement concerning the abdominal autonomic supply is *incorrect*?

- [ ] **a.** The coeliac ganglia receive fibres from the greater and lesser splanchnic nerves.
- [ ] **b.** The abdominal organs all derive their sympathetic supply from the coeliac ganglia.
- [ ] **c.** The greater splanchnic nerve contains fibres which innervate the adrenal cortex.
- [ ] **d.** The sympathetic system contains motor fibres to the sphincters.
- [ ] **e.** The pelvic splanchnic nerves contain parasympathetic fibres.

4.38 Which statement best describes the ureter?

- [ ] **a.** Is narrowest as it crosses the transverse process of L4.
- [ ] **b.** Is crossed anteriorly by the gonadal vessels.
- [ ] **c.** Is crossed anteriorly by the root of the mesentery on the left.
- [ ] **d.** It courses superior to the uterine vessels.
- [ ] **e.** Has a blood supply from the external iliac artery.

4.39 Which of the following structures does the ureter cross on an abdominal radiograph?

- [ ] **a.** The bodies of the lumbar vertebrae.
- [ ] **b.** Ischial tuberosity.
- [ ] **c.** Sacroiliac joint.
- [ ] **d.** Pubic tubercle.
- [ ] **e.** Tragal pointer.

ANSWERS

4.1

b. The transpyloric plane also passes through the pylorus, the pancreatic neck, the duodenojejunal flexure and the fundus of the gall bladder. The spinal cord also ends at the level of the transpyloric plane.

Explanations

a. The transpyloric plane (of Addison) lies halfway between the suprasternal notch and the symphysis pubis, approximately a hands breadth below the xiphoid. It is at the level of L1.

c. The subcostal plane is at the level of the body of L3 and joins the lowest point of the costal margin, the lower border of the 10th costal cartilage, of each side.

d. They lie at the level of L4. As the plane through the iliac crests lies well below the termination of the spinal cord it is a landmark used in performing a lumbar puncture. The tubercle of the ilium lies at the level of L5.

e. The umbilicus usually lies at the level of the L3/L4 disc. It is variable in position and lower in a gravid or obese abdomen.

4.2

a. The abdomen is conventionally divided into nine regions by the two mid-clavicular lines running vertically, and the transpyloric plane and intertubercular plane running horizontally. The intertubercular plane joins the tubercles of the iliac crests. The epigastrium is in the position described relative to these lines.

Explanations

b. The suprapubic region is below the intertubercular line and between the mid-clavicular lines.

c. The iliac fossa lies below the intertubercular line.

d. This describes the position of the umbilical region. The hypochondrium lies lateral to the mid-clavicular line and above the transpyloric plane.

e. The mid-clavicular line crosses the mid-inguinal point, which is half-way between the anterior superior iliac spine and the pubic symphysis. It is the surface marking of the femoral artery. This is distinct from the mid-point of the inguinal ligament, half-way between the anterior superior iliac spine and the pubic tubercle, which is the surface marking of the deep inguinal ring.

4.3

a. Camper's fascia is the superficial fatty layer of the fascia of the abdominal wall. This fatty layer is continuous with the fat of the rest of the body.

Explanations

b. Scarpa's fascia is the fibrous layer of the superficial fascia of the lower part of the abdominal wall. There is no deep fascia over the abdominal wall, allowing expansion during breathing.

c. Scarpa's fascia adheres to the deep fascia of the thigh (fascia lata), just below the skin crease. This explains why urine extravasated from a urethral injury extends up the abdominal wall, deep to Scarpa's fascia, rather than tracking down the leg.

d. The umbilicus is supplied by sensory fibres from T10.

e. The groin is supplied by fibres derived from L1. These run in the iliohypogastric and ilioinguinal nerves.

4.4

c. Below the arcuate line the aponeuroses of all three oblique muscles pass in front of the rectus abdominis. Above the arcuate line the external oblique aponeurosis passes anterior, the transverse oblique aponeurosis passes behind, and the internal oblique aponeurosis splits to enclose the rectus muscle.

Explanations

a. The transversalis fascia lies posterior along most of the length of the muscle. Above the costal margin, however, the 5th, 6th and 7th costal cartilages lie posteriorly.

b. The rectus abdominis has three tendinous intersections which are visible on the anterior surface of the muscle. They join the muscle to the rectus sheath at the umbilicus, the xiphoid and halfway in between. These intersections are not seen posteriorly so the rectus muscle is completely free behind at this level.

d. The arcuate line (of Douglas) lies halfway between the umbilicus and the pubis on the posterior surface of rectus abdominis. At the arcuate line the inferior epigastric vessels enter the rectus sheath and run up the posterior surface of the muscle.

e. The linea alba is a line joining the two halves of the rectus muscle. It is an avascular structure which can therefore be incised bloodlessly in a midline abdominal incision.

4.5

b. The lower border of the external oblique aponeurosis forms the inguinal ligament.

Explanations

a. The fibres of external oblique pass antero-inferiorly, the fibres of internal oblique pass antero-superiorly and the fibres of the transversus abdominis run transversely.

c. The external oblique arises from the lower eight ribs and inserts into the xiphoid, the linea alba, the pubis and the anterior half of the iliac crest.

d. The internal oblique arises from the lumbar fascia, the anterior 2/3 of the iliac crest and the lateral 2/3 of the inguinal ligament. It inserts into the lower six costal cartilages, the linea alba and the pubic crest.

e. This border consists of muscle fibres that lie in front of the spermatic cord laterally, behind it medially and above it in between. They are joined by fibres from transversus abdominis to form the conjoint tendon.

4.6

d. The conjoint tendon, comprising of the fused fibres of the internal and transverse oblique muscles, arches over the inguinal canal to attach to the pubic crest.

Explanations

a. The deep ring is a defect in the transversalis fascia.

b. The inguinal ligament is the lower border of the external oblique aponeurosis and forms the inferior border of the inguinal canal.

c. The internal oblique forms part of the anterior border of the inguinal canal laterally and then arches over the spermatic cord to form part of the posterior wall medially.

e. The ilioinguinal nerve enters the inguinal canal by passing through the internal oblique muscle. It runs anterior to the spermatic cord before leaving the canal through the superficial ring.

4.7

b. The greater omentum is formed by two double layers of peritoneum. The anterior two layers are continuous with the peritoneal layers enclosing the stomach. They then turn, double over and blend with the peritoneum of the transverse colon and mesocolon.

Explanations

a. The median umbilical fold is on the inner aspect of the anterior abdominal wall and contains the median umbilical ligament, which is the remnant of the obliterated urachus. The remnant of the umbilical artery is the medial umbilical ligament which lies within the medial umbilical fold. The lateral umbilical fold contains the inferior epigastric vessels.

c. The gastrosplenic ligament connects the greater curvature of the stomach to the spleen. It is a double layer of peritoneum containing the short gastric and left gastroepiploic vessels.

d. The lienorenal ligament connects the anterior surface of the left kidney to the spleen. It is a double layer of peritoneum containing the splenic vessels and the tail of the pancreas.

e. The lesser omentum connects the liver to the lesser curvature of the stomach and on to the commencement of the first part of the duodenum.

4.8

e. These ligamentous structures form the left border of the lesser sac.

Explanations

a. The greater sac is connected to the lesser sac via the epiploic foramen (of Winslow).

b. The anterior border of the lesser sac is formed by the lesser omentum, the peritoneum over the stomach and the greater omentum.

c. The posterior wall of the lesser sac is formed by the posterior layer of the greater omentum which adheres to the transverse colon and transverse mesocolon. Much of the posterior wall is made up of this layer of peritoneum covering the pancreas. This explains why fluid produced during pancreatitis can go on to form a pseudocyst at this location.

d. The anterior layer of the greater omentum forms part of the anterior border of the lesser sac.

4.9

e. The free border of the lesser omentum, which forms the anterior border, contains the hepatic artery and common bile duct anteriorly and the portal vein posteriorly. The hepatic artery is found on the left of the common bile duct. This arrangement of structures allows compression of the hepatic artery between finger and thumb (Pringle's manoeuvre) to control bleeding from the cystic artery and the liver.

Explanations

a. The inferior border of the epiploic foramen (of Winslow) is the first part of the duodenum.

b. The caudate process of the liver forms the superior border.

c. The inferior vena cava forms the posterior border of the epiploic foramen.

d. The right free border of the lesser omentum forms the anterior border.

4.10

c. This space communicates medially with the lesser sac via the epiploic foramen. The lateral border is the diaphragm. The superior border is the inferior border of the coronary ligament and the triangular ligament.

Explanations

a. The infracolic compartment lies below the attachment of the transverse mesocolon to the posterior abdominal wall, the supracolic compartment lies above it.

b. The subphrenic spaces are separated by the falciform ligament. The coronary ligament forms the superior border of the right subhepatic space. The left subhepatic space is closed superiorly by the left triangular ligament.

d. The left subhepatic space is the lesser sac. The hepatorenal pouch (of Rutherford–Morrison) is the right subhepatic space.

e. The right paracolic gutter is found lateral to the ascending colon.

4.11

b. The coeliac trunk arises from the aorta at the level of T12, a little below the median arcuate ligament.

Explanations

a. The coeliac trunk is the artery of the foregut and supplies the gut from the lower oesophagus to the opening of the duodenal papilla into the duodenum. It also supplies the liver, pancreas and spleen, which are derived from the foregut.

c. Branches of the left gastric artery supply the lower oesophagus by passing up through the oesophageal hiatus in the diaphragm.

d. The splenic artery is characteristically tortuous; this enables it to be readily identified at operation.

e. The hepatic artery has right gastric and gastroduodenal branches. The right gastric artery leaves the common hepatic artery and runs in the lesser omentum, supplying the stomach. The gastroduodenal artery further divides into a superior pancreaticoduodenal branch, which supplies the head of the pancreas and the duodenum, and the right gastroepiploic artery, which supplies the stomach. The close posterior relationship of the pancreaticoduodenal vessels to the duodenum explains the heavy bleeding that may occur from a posterior duodenal ulcer.

4.12

e. The short gastric arteries are variable in number. Most commonly six are present. They run in the gastrosplenic ligament to supply the lateral surface of the stomach.

Explanations

a. The blood supply of the stomach is derived from the three branches of the coeliac curvature: the left gastric, splenic and common hepatic arteries.

b. The gastroepiploic vessels run along the greater curvature of the stomach. The right is a branch of the gastroduodenal artery, which arises from the hepatic artery. The left is a branch of the splenic artery.

c. The right gastric artery is a branch of the common hepatic artery.

d. The left gastroepiploic artery arises from the hepatic artery.

4.13

c. The superior mesenteric vein passes over the uncinate process of the pancreas before joining the splenic vein behind its neck. It is trapped in this position by the fusion of the dorsal and ventral pancreatic diverticulae during development of the pancreas.

Explanations

a. Blood from the upper oesophagus and lower anal canal drains into the systemic circulation, forming portosystemic anastomoses. In portal hypertension varices can form at these sites, which can be liable to heavy bleeding.

b. The portal vein is formed by the union of the splenic and superior mesenteric veins behind the neck of the pancreas.

d. The inferior mesenteric vein passes in front of the left renal vein, before entering the splenic vein behind the body of the pancreas.

e. The prepyloric vein (of Mayo) is constant in its position over the pylorus in the stomach and can be used to identify this sphincter at operation. Most of the gastrointestinal tract is drained by veins which are named the same as their equivalent arteries. The gastroduodenal artery, however, has no equivalent vein.

4.14

b. The superior mesenteric artery arises from the aorta at the level of L1 and then descends. It then passes behind the splenic vein and the body of the pancreas.

Explanations

a. The superior mesenteric artery is the artery of the midgut, and supplies the duodenum, small intestine and the large intestine as far as a point 2/3 of the way along the transverse colon.

c. The superior mesenteric artery passes anterior to the uncinate process of the pancreas and the left renal vein.

d. The superior mesenteric vessels cross the third part of the duodenum after passing over the uncinate process of the pancreas.

e. The appendix is supplied by the appendicular branch of the iliocolic artery, which also supplies the ileocaecal junction and the caecum. The right colic artery supplies the ascending colon. The superior mesenteric artery also gives off jejunal and ileal branches, which supply the small intestine, and the middle colic artery, which supplies the transverse colon.

4.15

c. The left colic artery has ascending and descending branches. In a sigmoid colectomy the ascending branch is preserved to maintain the blood supply of the proximal descending colon.

Explanations

a. The inferior mesenteric artery arises from the aorta at the level of the subcostal plane, 3–4 cm above the aortic bifurcation. This is at the level of L3 and approximately at the level of the umbilicus.

b. The inferior mesenteric artery supplies the mucous membrane as far as the dentate line, which is found in the anus. This line represents a watershed between the superior rectal branch of the inferior mesenteric artery, and the middle and inferior rectal arteries which are derived from the internal iliac artery.

d. The inferior mesenteric artery enters the pelvis by crossing the pelvic brim at the level of bifurcation of the left common iliac artery.

e. The left colic branch anastomoses with the middle colic branch of the superior mesenteric artery. The other branches of the inferior mesenteric artery are the sigmoid arteries, supplying the sigmoid colon and the aforementioned superior rectal artery.

4.16
d. There are coeliac, superior mesenteric and inferior mesenteric groups of lymph nodes which lie around the origins of the major blood vessels and drain lymph from their territories of supply.

Explanations
a. The lymph vessels follow the venous drainage of the bowel. Therefore, if a segment of bowel is resected with its blood supply then the area of mesentery removed will include the local lymph nodes.

b. Peyer's patches are aggregations of lymphoid follicles in the ileum and lie on its antimesenteric surface.

c. Lymhoid follicles form the mucosa-associated lymphoid tissue (MALT) which lies along the entire gastrointestinal tract from mouth to anus. In the ileum they become aggregated into Peyer's patches. In the large bowel they are more numerous but isolated from each other.

e. The lymph from the gastrointestinal tract eventually drains into the cisterna chyli and then into the left brachiocephalic vein via the thoracic duct.

4.17
b. All the lymph drainage from the stomach eventually drains into the coeliac nodes and then into the cisterna chyli.

Explanations
a. The lymph from the stomach initially drains in three directions. On the right side the lymph drains to the left and right gastric nodes. On the left the superior portion drains into the pancreaticosplenic nodes and suprapancreatic nodes and the inferior portion drains into nodes around the pylorus.

c. The anterior and posterior vagi pass along the lesser curvature of the stomach and give off gastric branches as they descend.

d. The nerves of Latarjet (greater anterior and greater posterior gastric nerves) are large branches from the anterior and posterior vagi. These nerves run in the lesser omentum to reach the pylorus, which they supply. The operation of highly selective vagotomy aims to preserve these nerves while dividing the gastric branches, preserving the nerve supply to the pylorus and removing the need to perform a drainage procedure.

e. Hydrochloric acid is secreted by parietal cells in the body of the stomach. In the antrum mucus secreting cells are joined by gastrin secreting G cells and D cells which produce somatostatin.

4.18

c. The ampulla of Vater opens into the second part of the duodenum. It opens onto an eminence called the duodenal papilla which is formed by the union of the common bile duct and pancreatic duct.

Explanations

a. The second part of the duodenum curves around the head of the pancreas and lies on the right kidney and ureter. It is therefore at the risk of damage in operations on the right kidney.

b. The attachment of the transverse mesocolon lies over the second part. The upper half of the duodenum is therefore in the supracolic compartment and the lower half is in the infracolic compartment.

d. The third part of the duodenum runs transversely as a continuation of the second part. It crosses the inferior vena cava and aorta anterior to L3. It is crossed anteriorly by the superior mesenteric vessels.

e. This relationship allows ulceration of a gallstone into the duodenum, which may result in gallstone ileus.

4.19

a. The jejunum has thicker walls than the ileum as the valvulae conniventes are larger proximally.

Explanations

b. The proximal small intestine is of greater diameter.

c. The mesentery becomes thicker and has more fat more distally.

d. The jejunum usually lies in the umbilical region, the ileum lies in the hypogastrium and pelvis.

e. The mesenteric vessels form one or two arcades in the jejunum and four to five arcades in the ileum.

4.20

b. Meckel's diverticulum represents the proximal remnant of the embryonic yolk stalk, and as such is found at the site of attachment of the yolk stalk at the border of the intestine opposite its mesenteric attachment.

Explanations

a. It is an ileal congenital anomaly which is found in approximately 2% of the population, it is the embryological remnant of the vitellointestinal duct. Meckel's diverticulum is of clinical significance as it may become inflamed and mimic the presentation of an acute appendicitis or cause rectal bleeding.

c. It is usually about 5 cm (2 inch.) in length. A commonly quoted statement about Meckel's diverticulum is that it is present in 2% of the population, 2 ft from the ileocaecal junction and is 2 inch. in length.

d. It is usually found 40 cm from the ileocaecal junction in children, and at about 60 cm in adults.

e. At the apex the diverticulum may be directly adherent to, or connected by, a fibrous cord to the umbilicus. In 75% of people, however, it is free from attachment to the umbilicus.

4.21

d. The appendix is very variable in position. It may lie in a retro-ileal or pre-ileal (5%), retrocolic or retrocaecal (75%), subcaecal or pelvic (20%) position. Its variable position explains the huge range of differential diagnoses of appendicitis.

Explanations

a. The taenia coli, which run along the large bowel, are all attached at the base of the appendix. The appendix can therefore be identified by tracing these bands.

b. These vessels must be ligated in an appendicectomy.

c. The appendix, or the caecum, is connected to the ileum by this fold of peritoneum. Although also known as the bloodless fold of Treves, this fold often contains a blood vessel, which must be ligated during appendicectomy to achieve haemostasis.

e. The appendix opens into the posteromedial part of the caecum.

4.22

c. The hepatic flexure is directly in contact with the liver and the right kidney; it is therefore at risk in a right nephrectomy.

Explanations

a. The majority of the colon is derived from the midgut, which extends to a point just proximal to the splenic flexure. The descending colon and sigmoid are derived from the hindgut.

b. The ascending and descending colon are usually in contact with the abdominal wall posteriorly and with peritoneum on the rest of the surface. The posterior part is therefore free from peritoneum.

d. In foetal life the entire colon has a primitive hindgut mesentery. The ascending and descending colon lose this mesentery and become secondarily retroperitoneal. In some specimens the ascending and descending colon do not come into contact with the posterior abdominal wall and the primitive hindgut mesentery persists. This occurs in 10% of subjects in the ascending colon and 20% in the descending colon.

e. The appendices epiploicae are pouches of peritoneum which are filled with fat.

4.23

c. The sigmoid colon hangs free on the sigmoid mesocolon.

Explanations

a. The taenia coli are shorter than the colon and represent its longitudinal muscle. Their short length causes the colon to become sacculated.

b. The transverse colon is the longest part of the large bowel. It is approximately 45 cm long. The descending colon is less than 30 cm long; the ascending colon is 15 cm long and the sigmoid slightly less than 45 cm. These lengths are variable.

d. The vagus nerve supplies the large bowel with parasympathetic fibres as far as the junction of the primitive mid- and hindguts. The hindgut is supplied with parasympathetic fibres via the pelvic splanchnic nerves.

e. The marginal artery runs within the mesentery adjacent to the bowel. The marginal artery (of Drummond) is the name given to the anastomotic branches which join the arterial arcades along the whole bowel.

4.24

d. The abdominal oesophagus grooves the posterior aspect of the left lobe of the liver.

Explanations

a. The structures on the inferior surface of the liver form an H-shape. The cross bar of the H is the porta hepatis. The anterior two bars are the fissure for the gall bladder on the right and the fissure for the ligamentum teres on the left. The posterior two bars are the inferior vena cava on the right and the ligamentum venosum on the left. The ligamentum venosum therefore lies posterior and to the left of the gall bladder.

b. The falciform ligament contains the ligamentum teres in its inferior free border. The ligamentum teres is the obliterated remnant of the left umbilical vein.

c. The quadrate lobe lies anteriorly between the anterior two bars of the H and the caudate lobe lies posteriorly between the two posterior bars.

e. The anatomical lobes of the liver are separated by the plane between the ligamentum venosum and the falciform ligament. The vascular supply of the liver demarcates the morphological left and right lobes differently. The functional (or morphological) lobes are separated by a line drawn through the fossae for the gall bladder and inferior vena cava.

4.25

d. The parasympathetic fibres that supply the liver run in the vagus nerve.

Explanations

a. The hepatic artery lies between the common hepatic duct and the portal vein, in the middle of the porta hepatis.

b. The common hepatic artery lies anteriorly, making it the most accessible structure surgically.

c. The portal vein is the most posterior structure in the porta hepatis.

e. The liver is a derivative of the primitive foregut and therefore the sympathetic supply follows the blood supply from the coeliac plexus.

4.26

e. Branches of the left and right colic and splenic veins, which drain into the portal system, anastomose with small retroperitoneal veins, which drain into renal, lumbar and phrenic veins.

Explanations

a. The portal vein is formed by the union of the splenic and superior mesenteric veins. The inferior mesenteric vein empties into the splenic vein. The portal vein drains the abdominal gastrointestinal tract.

b. At the anal canal there is an anastomosis between the superior rectal veins, which drain into the portal system via the inferior mesenteric vein, and the middle veins, which drain into the inferior vena cava. Rectal varices may, therefore, form in portal hypertension.

c. The lower third of the oesophagus is drained inferiorly into the portal system by oesophageal branches of the left gastric vein. Superiorly it is drained by oesophageal veins, which empty into the azygos and hemiazygos systems. In portal hypertension varices form at this site of anastomosis and may bleed, causing severe haemetemesis.

d. Paraumbilical veins which pass along the falciform ligament to drain into the left branch of the portal vein, anastomose with the epigastric veins of the anterior abdominal wall.

4.27

a. The bare area of the liver lies between the anterior and posterior layers of the coronary ligament. These two layers meet in a sharp point on the right, which is known as the right triangular ligament. The left triangular ligament is formed from the left leaf of the falciform ligament.

Explanations

b. The coronary ligament is continuous with the right leaf of the falciform ligament.

c. The bare area is a triangle formed by the two leaves of the coronary ligament, which meet as the right triangular ligament on the right side. The base of the triangle is formed by the inferior vena cava on the left.

d. The structures of the porta hepatis run in the free edge of the lesser omentum, which forms the anterior border of the epiploic foramen.

e. The bare area is related to the right suprarenal gland and the diaphragm.

4.28

d. The common bile duct may be described in three portions. The first part lies in the free edge of the lesser omentum. The second part lies behind the first part of the duodenum.

Explanations

a. The pancreatic duct drains into the duodenum via a common opening with the common bile duct.

b. The cystic duct joins the common hepatic duct to form the common bile duct.

c. Callot's triangle is formed by the common hepatic duct, cystic duct and the edge of the liver. The cystic artery usually runs through this triangle. The significant variations in biliary anatomy mean that all components of the triangle must be identified before the cystic artery and cystic duct can be safely ligated during cholecystectomy.

e. The third part of the common bile duct lies in a groove between the second part of the duodenum and the back of the head of the pancreas, which it grooves.

4.29

c. The kidneys are related to the posterior abdominal wall muscles: psoas major, quadratus lumborum and the transversus abdominis muscle.

Explanations

a. The suprarenals lie above the kidneys on both sides.

b. The duodenum is related to the anteromedial part of the right kidney. The duodenum is not related to the left kidney.

d. The pancreas is related to the left kidney below the stomach and above the small bowel.

e. The hepatic flexure of the transverse colon is related to the right kidney.

4.30

b. This thin layer of fascia blends with that over the inferior vena cava and aorta.

Explanations

a. The suprarenals are contained in a separate fascial compartment. This enables them to be easily separated from the kidney at nephrectomy.

c. The perinephric fat lies within the renal fascia.

d. The lienorenal ligament connects the left kidney with the spleen. It contains the splenic vessels.

e. The true capsule of the kidney lies between the kidney and the perirenal fascia and covers the kidney beneath the perinephric fat.

4.31

a. The neck lies in the transpyloric plane at the level of L1.

Explanations

b. The splenic artery runs behind the pancreas and give branches which supply it. The arteria pancreatica magna is the name given to the largest branch.

c. The uncinate process drains its secretions through the accessory pancreatic duct (of Santorini) into the second part of the duodenum, a little above the ampulla.

d. The relationship of the head of the pancreas to the second part of the duodenum is exploited in Kocher's manoeuvre, in which an incision is made along the peritoneum lateral to the duodenum, allowing the duodenum and head of the pancreas to be mobilised anteriorly.

e. The pancreas develops from ventral and dorsal buds which arise from the foregut. The uncinate process is derived from the anterior bud and the body from the posterior bud. The anterior bud of the pancreas swings anteriorly and traps the superior mesenteric vessels inferiorly.

4.32

a. The anterior border of the spleen is notched, it is said that this allows an enlarged spleen to be identified during abdominal examination.

Explanations

b. This is correct.

c. The left kidney and stomach are both direct relations of the spleen. It is therefore at risk in a left nephrectomy.

d. The spleen is completely enclosed in peritoneum, derived form the dorsal mesogastrium.

e. The pancreas abuts the spleen at this point and must be carefully protected during splenectomy.

4.33

e. The medial arcuate ligament is a condensation of the thick psoas fascia. The sympathetic trunk passes under this ligament to enter the abdomen.

Explanations

a. The femoral nerve emerges lateral to psoas major. It is a branch of the lumbar plexus, the divisions of which lie within the muscle. The subcostal, iliohypogastric, ilioinguinal, lateral femoral cutaneous and femoral nerves traverse the muscle to emerge at the lateral border.

b. The obturator nerve emerges medial to psoas major and runs down to the obturator foramen, which it passes through to gain access to the medial compartment of the thigh.

c. The genitofemoral nerve pierces psoas major and emerges on its anterior surface.

d. It is attached distally to the lesser trochanter of the femur. Its action is to flex the thigh at the hip.

4.34

a. The abdominal aorta gives four paired lumbar branches which supply the body wall and spine. The 5th lumbar arteries are derived from the iliolumbar arteries, which are branches of the posterior divisions of the internal iliac arteries. The four midline branches of the aorta are the coeliac trunk (T12), superior mesenteric artery (L1), inferior mesenteric artery (L3) and the median sacral artery. There are three pairs of visceral branches: the suprarenal, renal (L2) and gonadal arteries.

Explanations

b. The body of the pancreas crosses the abdominal aorta between the origins of the coeliac trunk and the superior mesenteric artery, as does the splenic vein. The left renal vein, the uncinate process of the pancreas and the third part of the duodenum cross the aorta between the origin of the superior and inferior mesenteric vessels.

c. The first branch of the abdominal aorta is the inferior phrenic artery. The subcostal artery is the lowest branch of the thoracic aorta and enters the abdomen beneath the lateral arcuate ligament.

d. The aorta ends at the level of the L4 vertebra. This is at the level of the supracristal line and equates to a point approximately 2.5 cm below the umbilicus.

e. The suprarenals are each supplied by three arteries. The superior is derived from a twig from the inferior phrenic arteries (the first branch of the abdominal aorta), the middle is derived directly from the abdominal aorta and the inferior is a branch of the renal artery.

4.35

e. The hepatic veins drain into the inferior vena cava as it passes behind the liver.

Explanations

a. The inferior vena cava is formed by the union of the common iliac veins at the level of L5.

b. The veins draining the gastrointestinal tract drain into the portal system, not into the inferior vena cava.

c. The second lumbar vein, as well as the first lumbar vein, joins the ascending lumbar vein. The bottom three lumbar veins are tributaries of the inferior vena cava.

d. The subcostal vein joins the ascending lumbar vein to form the azygos vein on the right and the hemiazygos vein on the left.

4.36

b. They are both derived from L1. The ilioinguinal nerve represents the collateral branch of the iliohypogastric nerve. The iliohypogastric nerve supplies suprapubic skin, the ilioinguinal nerve supplies the anterior 1/3 of the scrotum/labium majus and the root of the penis/clitoris.

Explanations

a. The lumbar plexus is formed by the primary rami of L1–L4. They give segmental branches which supply quadratus lumborum and psoas and then divide into anterior and posterior divisions, which form the lumbar plexus within the substance of the muscle.

c. The femoral nerve is derived from the posterior divisions of the anterior rami of L2–L4. The obturator nerve is derived from the anterior divisions of the anterior primary rami.

d. The genital branch of the genitofemoral nerve traverses the inguinal canal. It gives motor fibres to the cremaster muscle, sensory fibres to the covering of the cord and sensory fibres to the area of scrotal skin not supplied by the ilioinguinal nerve.

e. Part of the anterior primary ramus of L4 and L5 join to form the lumbosacral trunk which contributes to the sacral plexus.

4.37

c. Preganglionic fibres pass from the greater splanchnic nerve to supply the adrenal medulla. Stimulation of these fibres causes secretion of catecholamines into the circulation.

Explanations

a. The greater and lesser splanchnic nerves carry preganglionic fibres which run down to the coeliac ganglia where they synapse.

b. The fibres from the coeliac ganglia spread down the aorta and follow the blood vessels to their target organs. The pelvic organs receive their sympathetic innervation via the superior and inferior hypogastric plexi.

d. The sympathetic nervous system acts to cause contraction of the abdominal sphincters, for example, the pylorus.

e. The pelvic splanchnic nerves are derived from the anterior primary rami of S2–S4. They carry parasympathetic fibres to the pelvic organs and the gastrointestinal tract distal to the splenic flexure.

4.38

b. The gonadal vessels cross the ureter anteriorly.

Explanations

a. The ureter has three narrow points: as it arises from the renal pelvis, as it crosses the pelvic brim and as it enters the bladder. The first of these is the tightest. These points are clinically important because they represent the likely site of impaction of a renal stone.

c. The root of the mesentery crosses the ureter on the right side.

d. The ureter courses inferior to the uterine vessels which run in the inferior edge of the broad ligament. It is therefore at risk in a hysterectomy.

e. The ureter derives its blood supply from the vessels with which it comes into contact: the renal artery, the abdominal aorta, the gonadal vessels, the common and internal iliac arteries, the superior vesicular and the uterine arteries. This blood supply is at risk if the surrounding tissue is stripped from the ureter. The external iliac artery does not supply the ureter as it is not related to it.

4.39

c. The ureter crosses the pelvic brim over the sacroiliac joint.

Explanations

a. The ureter lies over the transverse processes of the lumbar vertebrae on an abdominal film.

b. The ureter turns medially to enter the bladder over the ischial spine, not the ischial tuberosity.

d. The ureter passes into the bladder along the line between the ischial spine and the pubic tubercle, but stops short of overlying it.

e. The tragal pointer is a landmark for the facial nerve.

5

Pelvis

QUESTIONS

5.1 Which of the following statements best describes the bony pelvis?

- [ ] **a.** The true pelvis lies between the iliac crests.
- [ ] **b.** The acetabulum is formed by contributions from all parts of the inominate bone.
- [ ] **c.** The male pelvic inlet has a more oval shape than in the female.
- [ ] **d.** The angle between the inferior pubic rami is wider in the male.
- [ ] **e.** The pelvic outlet is between the symphysis pubis and the sacral tuberosity.

5.2 Which of the following statements about the ligaments of the pelvis is *incorrect*?

- [ ] **a.** The inguinal ligament passes from the anterior superior iliac spine to the pubic tubercle.
- [ ] **b.** The sacrospinous ligament is a border of the lesser sciatic foramen.
- [ ] **c.** The sacrotuberous ligament is a border of the lesser sciatic foramen.
- [ ] **d.** The lacunar ligament forms the lateral border of the femoral canal.
- [ ] **e.** The sacrospinous ligament provides an attachment for coccygeus.

5.3 Which of the following associations of joints and types is correct?

- ☐ **a.** Symphysis pubis   Primary cartilaginous
- ☐ **b.** Sacroiliac joint   Synovial
- ☐ **c.** Lumbosacral joint   Primary cartilaginous
- ☐ **d.** Acetabulofemoral   Fibrous
- ☐ **e.** Sacrococcygeal   Fibrous

5.4 Which of the following structures does *not* pass through the greater sciatic foramen?

- ☐ **a.** Piriformis.
- ☐ **b.** Sciatic nerve.
- ☐ **c.** Superior gluteal nerve.
- ☐ **d.** Inferior gluteal nerve.
- ☐ **e.** Gemellus superior.

5.5 Which of the following structures passes through the lesser sciatic foramen?

- ☐ **a.** The posterior cutaneous nerve of the thigh.
- ☐ **b.** The pudendal nerve.
- ☐ **c.** Obturator externus.
- ☐ **d.** Gemellus superior.
- ☐ **e.** Gemellus inferior.

5.6 Which statement most correctly completes the following sentence? Levator ani:

- ☐ **a.** Attaches to the fascia over obturator internus.
- ☐ **b.** Has fibres which assist continence by pulling the rectum posteriorly.
- ☐ **c.** Lies inferior to the ischiorectal fossa.
- ☐ **d.** Is supplied by anterior primary rami of S1 and S2.
- ☐ **e.** Contracts during defaecation.

5.7 Which statement about the perineum is the correct one?

☐ **a.** It is divided by a line drawn between the ischial spines.

☐ **b.** The perineal body lies between the anterior and posterior parts of the perineum.

☐ **c.** The perineal membrane lies in the posterior part of the perineum.

☐ **d.** Bartholin's glands lie deep to the perineal membrane.

☐ **e.** The posterior part of the perineum is bounded laterally by the sacrospinous ligaments.

5.8 Which statement about the rectum and its relations is *incorrect*?

☐ **a.** There are two rectal folds on the left.

☐ **b.** The anorectal junction is related to the puborectalis muscle.

☐ **c.** The upper 1/3 is entirely invested in peritoneum.

☐ **d.** The pararectal lymph nodes lie in the mesorectum.

☐ **e.** Denonvillier's fascia lies below the rectovesical pouch.

5.9 Which statement best describes the anus and its sphincters?

☐ **a.** The anus contains longitudinal and circular muscle.

☐ **b.** The external sphincter is composed of involuntary muscle.

☐ **c.** The external sphincter is continuous with the muscle of the rectum.

☐ **d.** The anorectal ring is formed by puborectalis.

☐ **e.** The anal cushions are found in the left lateral, right posterior and right anterior positions.

5.10 Which statement best describes the bladder?

☐ **a.** The interureteric bar joins the two ureteric orifices.

☐ **b.** The venous drainage follows the course of the arterial supply.

☐ **c.** It has a blood supply principally derived from the external iliac artery.

☐ **d.** It is lined by specialised non-keratinising squamous epithelium.

☐ **e.** The sensation of bladder fullness is conveyed by sympathetic fibres.

5.11 Which statement best describes the pelvic viscera?

☐ **a.** The vas deferens is formed by the union of the ejaculatory ducts and the seminal vesicles.

☐ **b.** The vas deferens runs through the inguinal canal.

☐ **c.** The vas deferens passes anterior to the urethra to enter the bladder.

☐ **d.** The ejaculatory ducts enter the spongy urethra.

☐ **e.** The bulbourethral glands enter the prostatic urethra.

5.12 Which statement about the prostate is *incorrect*?

☐ **a.** The urethal crest is found on the posterior wall of the urethra.

☐ **b.** It lies between the bladder and the external urethral sphincter.

☐ **c.** The urethra runs through the posterior part of the gland.

☐ **d.** It may have a true and a false capsule.

☐ **e.** It is supplied by the inferior vesical arteries.

5.13 Which statement regarding the male perineum is *incorrect*?

☐ **a.** The root of the penis is attached to the perineal membrane.

☐ **b.** The membranous urethra lies superficial to the perineal membrane.

☐ **c.** Cowper's glands lie deep to the perineal membrane.

☐ **d.** Colles' fascia is attached to the perineal membrane.

☐ **e.** The sphincter urethrae contains voluntary muscle.

5.14 Which statement best describes the spermatic cord?

☐ **a.** The internal spermatic fascia is derived from the transversus abdominis muscle.

☐ **b.** The cremasteric fascia contains muscle fibres derived from external oblique.

☐ **c.** It contains the genital branch of the genitofemoral nerve.

☐ **d.** It contains the ilioinguinal nerve.

☐ **e.** It contains the testicular vein.

5.15 Which statement best describes the testis and epididymis?

☐ **a.** The vas deferens arises from the upper pole of the epididymis.

☐ **b.** The appendix testis is attached to the lower pole of the testis.

☐ **c.** The tunica vaginalis lies deep to the tunica albuginea.

☐ **d.** The testis is divided into lobules by septa.

☐ **e.** The dartos muscle lies deep to the cremasteric fascia.

5.16 Which statement concerning the penis is *incorrect*?

☐ **a.** The corpora cavernosa are ensheathed by the tunica albuginea.

☐ **b.** The penile urethra runs within the corpus spongiosum.

☐ **c.** There are two deep penile arteries.

☐ **d.** Erection is under sympathetic control.

☐ **e.** Bulbospongiosus is important in micturition.

5.17 Which statement about the uterus and fallopian tubes is correct?

☐ **a.** The fundus lies posterior to the entrance of the fallopian tubes into the uterus.

☐ **b.** The cornu is the point of junction of the body of the uterus and the vagina.

☐ **c.** The ampulla of the fallopian tubes bare fimbrae.

☐ **d.** The fallopian tubes contain smooth muscle.

☐ **e.** The upper part drains lymph to the external iliac nodes.

5.18 Which of the following statements about the uterus is *incorrect*?

☐ **a.** The uterus is retroverted in 1/5 of nulliparous females.

☐ **b.** The uterine artery courses down the lateral wall of the uterus.

☐ **c.** The cervix is attached to the bladder.

☐ **d.** Develops from the paramesonephric ducts.

☐ **e.** The cardinal ligament is traversed by the ureter.

5.19 Which statement concerning the ovary is the correct one?

☐ **a.** The ovarian ligament contains the ovarian vessels.

☐ **b.** The right ovarian vein drains into the right renal vein.

☐ **c.** The suspensory ligament of the ovary is attached to the sidewall of the pelvis.

☐ **d.** Lymphatics drain to the internal iliac nodes.

☐ **e.** It is attached to the anterior aspect of the broad ligament.

5.20 Which structure is *not* contained within, or attached to, the broad ligament?

- ☐ **a.** The suspensory ligament of the ovary.
- ☐ **b.** The round ligament.
- ☐ **c.** The uterine artery.
- ☐ **d.** The fallopian tube.
- ☐ **e.** The ovarian ligament.

5.21 Which statement best describes the cervix and vagina?

- ☐ **a.** The anterior part of the cervix is covered with peritoneum.
- ☐ **b.** The vagina is covered with peritoneum anteriorly.
- ☐ **c.** The ureter is a close relation of the cervix.
- ☐ **d.** The entire vagina is supplied with sensory fibres by the pudendal nerve.
- ☐ **e.** The majority of the lymph from the vagina drains to the superficial inguinal nodes.

5.22 Which statement about the pelvic vasculature is correct?

- ☐ **a.** The common iliac artery divides over the sacro-iliac joint.
- ☐ **b.** The external iliac artery divides into anterior and posterior branches.
- ☐ **c.** The ovarian artery is a branch of the internal iliac artery.
- ☐ **d.** The inferior epigastric artery is a branch of the internal iliac artery.
- ☐ **e.** The obturator artery is a branch of the external iliac artery.

5.23 Which statement regarding the nerve supply of micturition is true?

- [ ] **a.** Contraction of the detrusor muscle is initiated by fibres from the inferior hypogastric plexus.
- [ ] **b.** The sphincter urethrae is innervated by the parasympathetic system.
- [ ] **c.** The internal urethral sphincter is parasympathetically innervated.
- [ ] **d.** Pubovaginalis helps to maintain continence in the female.
- [ ] **e.** Following a lumbar cord transection, bladder voiding is impossible.

5.24 Which statement does *not* correctly complete this sentence? The pudendal nerve:

- [ ] **a.** Enters the pelvis through the lesser sciatic foramen.
- [ ] **b.** Runs in a canal formed by the obturator internus fascia.
- [ ] **c.** Has a dorsal branch which is sensory to the penis.
- [ ] **d.** Has a perineal branch which is sensory to the clitoris.
- [ ] **e.** Gives motor fibres to the muscles of the urogenital diaphragm.

ANSWERS

5.1

b. The acetabulum is formed by contributions from the ilium, the ischium and the pubic bones.

Explanations

a. This statement defines the false pelvis, the true pelvis is the region inferior to the pelvic inlet.

c. The male pelvic inlet is heart shaped and the female is oval shaped. This helps to form a wide enough birth canal for the foetal head.

d. This angle is usually described as being the same as that between the forefinger and middle finger in the male, and between the thumb and forefinger in the female.

e. The pelvic inlet lies between the sacral tuberosity and the symphysis pubis. The pelvic outlet lies between the symphysis pubis and the coccyx.

5.2

d. The femoral canal is bounded by the femoral vein laterally, the lacunar ligament medially, the inguinal ligament anteriorly and the pectineal ligament posteriorly.

Explanations

a. It passes from the anterior superior iliac spine to the pubic tubercle.

b. The sacrospinous ligament passes from the anterior border of the sacrum to the ischial spine and forms the superior border of the lesser sciatic foramen.

c. The sacrotuberous ligament passes from the sacrum to the ischial tuberosity and forms the lower border of the lesser sciatic foramen.

e. The sacrospinous ligament provides an attachment for coccygeus. Piriformis originates from the anterior part of the sacrum, passes through the greater sciatic foramen and inserts on the greater trochanter of the femur.

5.3

b. The sacroiliac joint is a plane synovial joint, which unusually contains fibrocartilage on the ilium. A typical synovial joint is characterised by bone ends covered by hyaline cartilage and surrounded by a capsule reinforced by ligaments and lined by synovial membrane. Synovial joints are capable of movement. In atypical synovial joints the bone ends are lined by fibrocartilage.

Explanations

a. The symphysis pubis is a secondary cartilaginous joint, as are most joints in the midline. A primary cartilaginous joint is one in which bone and hyaline cartilage meet. A secondary cartilaginous joint is a junction between bones covered by a laminar of hyaline cartilage, which are then joined by fibrocartilage.

c. The lumbosacral joint is secondary cartilaginous as are all other intervertebral joints.

d. The hip joint is a synovial ball and socket joint.

e. The sacrococcygeal joint is a secondary cartilaginous joint, it has this in common with all intervertebral joints. A fibrous joint occurs where bones are separated only by connective tissue and very little movement occurs. A good example is the sutures of the skull.

5.4

e. The gamelli take origin from the outer side of the lesser sciatic foramen, after which they join obturator internus to insert onto the posterior aspect of the femur.

Explanations

a. Piriformis passes through the greater sciatic foramen from its origin on the anterior aspect of the sacrum to insert onto the greater trochanter of the femur.

b. The sciatic nerve exits the pelvis and passes below piriformis into the posterior compartment of the thigh.

c. The superior gluteal nerve (L4, L5, S1) passes above piriformis, between gluteus medius and gluteus minimus, which it supplies.

d. The inferior gluteal nerve (L5, S1, S2) passes below piri-formis to supply gluteus maximus.

5.5

b. The pudendal nerve (S2, S3, S4) arises from the sacral plexus. It exits the pelvis through the greater sciatic foramen and then re-enters through the lesser sciatic foramen. It runs in Alcock's canal and gives motor and sensory branches to structures in the perineum.

Explanations

a. The posterior cutaneous nerve of the thigh exits the pelvis through the greater sciatic foramen and the runs on the posterior aspect of the sciatic nerve. It innervates the skin on the back of the thigh as far as the popliteal fossa.

c. Obturator internus passes through the lesser sciatic foramen to its insertion on the greater trochanter of the femur.

d. Gemellus superior arises from the spine of the ischium and inserts onto the greater trochanter of the femur. It runs above obturator internus.

e. Gemellus inferior arises from the ischial tuberosity and inserts onto the greater trochanter of the femur. It runs below the obturator internus.

5.6

a. Levator ani is attached to the condensation of the fascia overlying obturator internus, known as the tendinous arch.

Explanations

b. The puborectalis fibres of levator ani arise from the back of the pubic bone and pass around the anorectal junction. They assist continence by pulling the rectum anteriorly.

c. The ischiorectal fossa is a fat filled space which lies inferior to levator ani and lateral to the rectum.

d. Levator ani is supplied by the anterior primary rami of S3 and S4.

e. Levator ani relaxes during defaecation to allow the rectum to straighten.

5.7

b. The perineal body is a mass of fibromuscular tissue which lies in the midline between the ischial tuberosities. It provides attachment sites for the perineal muscles.

Explanations

a. The perineum is a diamond-shaped area bounded by the symphysis pubis, ischial tuberosities and the coccyx. It is considered in an anterior and posterior triangle separated by an imaginary line drawn between the ischial tuberosities.

c. The perineal membrane is a sheet of connective tissue which lies in the anterior, urogenital region of the perineum. It is attached to the pubic rami and provides attachment for the root of the penis and the superficial perineal muscles.

d. Bartholin's glands lie superficial to the perineal membrane. This is in contrast with their male equivalent, Cowper's glands, which lie deep to the membrane. A Bartholin's abscess can therefore be drained through the skin.

e. The anal region of the perineum is bounded laterally by the sacrotuberous ligaments.

5.8

c. The upper 1/3 of the rectum is covered by peritoneum at the front and sides only. The middle third is covered in peritoneum only at the front. The lower third of the rectum has no peritoneal covering.

Explanations

a. The rectal folds, or rectal valves of Houston, are the internal marking of the lateral curves or flexures of the rectum. There are two on the left and one on the right.

b. The puborectalis muscle, the innermost fibres of levator ani, slings around the anorectal junction and pulls it anteriorly, helping to maintain continence.

d. The mesorectum is, strictly speaking, a condensation of the pelvic visceral fascia and is not derived from the true foetal mesentery. The pararectal lymph nodes lie within this layer, necessitating its removal in excision of a rectal carcinoma.

e. The rectovesical pouch is formed by a reflection of the peritoneum from the anterior surface of the rectum onto the bladder. Below the peritoneum the bladder is separated from the rectum in the male by a condensation of connective tissue called the rectovesical fascia, or the fascia of Denonvilliers. There is a similar fascial plane in the female between the rectum and the posterior aspect of the vagina.

5.9

d. Muscle fibres from puborectalis fuse with the muscle fibres of the external anal sphincter to form a ring of muscle, the anorectal ring, which is palpable on digital rectal examination.

Explanations

a. In contrast to the rest of the gut all of the muscle fibres of the anus are circular; they are arranged into an external and internal sphincter.

b. The external sphincter is made up of voluntary muscle supplied by the pudendal nerve. The internal sphincter is composed of involuntary muscle.

c. The internal sphincter is continuous with the inner circular muscle of the rectum.

e. The inverse is true. The anal cushions are composed of fibroelastic connective tissue, an arteriovenous anastomosis and smooth muscle. They classically lie in the right lateral, left posterior and left anterior positions. When viewed in the lithotomy position this is often referred to as the "3, 7 and 11 o'clock positions".

5.10

a. The interureteric bar is a thickening of muscle visible at cystoscopy as the interureteric ridge. This helps in the location of the ureteric orifices.

Explanations

b. The veins of the bladder form a plexus of veins and do not follow the arterial supply. This venous plexus eventually drains into the internal iliac veins.

c. The bladder is supplied by superior and inferior vesical arteries, which are branches of the anterior division of the internal iliac artery.

d. The bladder, along with the rest of the urinary tract, is lined by transitional epithelium, hence the common occurrence of transitional cell carcinomas in this region.

e. The sensation of bladder fullness is conveyed with parasympathetic fibres and courses up the spinal cord in the gracile tract.

5.11

b. The ejaculatory duct is formed by the union of the seminal vesicles and the vas deferens.

Explanations

b. The vas deferens runs through the inguinal canal within the spermatic cord.

c. The vas deferens runs anterior to the ureter to enter the prostate.

d. They enter the prostatic urethra at the level of the urethral crest on either side of the prostatic utricle.

e. The bulbourethral, or Cowper's, glands enter the spongy urethra. They lie in the deep perineal pouch and make a small contribution to the seminal fluid.

5.12

c. The urethra passes through the anterior part of the gland. There is more prostatic tissue behind the urethra than in front of it.

Explanations

a. The urethral crest lies on the posterior urethra as a longitudinal elevation. It bears the colliculus semilunaris as a prominence in the midline. The prostatic utricle opens from the middle of the verumontanum (colliculus semilunaris). The ejaculatory ducts open on either side of the utricle.

b. The external urethral sphincter (sphincter urethrae) ensheathes the membranous urethra and part of the prostatic urethra.

d. The true capsule of the prostate is composed of fibrous tissue and surrounds the gland directly. The false capsule is pathological and is composed of condensed normal prostatic tissue around the fibroglandular enlarged prostatic tissue.

e. The inferior vesical arteries are branches of the anterior division of the internal iliac arteries.

5.13
b. The membranous urethra lies deep to the perineal membrane between it and the prostate. Once it emerges superficial through the membrane, the prostatic urethra becomes the penile urethra.

Explanations
a. The root of the penis is attached to the perineal membrane. It consists of two crura and the bulb.

c. Cowper's glands lie on either side of the membranous urethra and contribute a small amount to the seminal fluid.

d. Colles' fascia is the perineal continuation of the fibrous layer of abdominal superficial fascia (Scarpa's fascia). It is attached to the posterior part of the perineal membrane. Urine extravasated from a ruptured membranous urethra tracks under Colles' fascia, and may, therefore, distend the scrotum and penis.

e. The sphinchter urethrae is made up of slow twitch striated muscle fibres, which surround the membranous urethra and extend upwards to ensheath part of the prostatic urethra.

5.14
c. This nerve supplies the cremaster muscle.

Explanations
a. The internal spermatic fascia is derived from the transversalis fascia at the deep inguinal ring. The fascia is "picked up" by the testis as it descends through the inguinal canal into the scrotum.

b. These fibres, which make up the cremasteric fascia, are derived from internal oblique. The external spermatic fascia is derived from the external oblique.

d. Strictly speaking the ilioinguinal nerve lies on, not within, the spermatic cord. It also enters the canal separately and not through the deep ring.

e. The testicular vein is formed from the pampiniform plexus, a network of veins within the spermatic cord, at the deep inguinal ring, proximal to the spermatic cord.

5.15

d. The testis is divided into approximately 200 lobules by fibrous septa. Each lobule contains three or four seminiferous tubules.

Explanations

a. The vas deferens arises from the lower pole of the epididymis, before ascending in the spermatic cord to enter the inguinal canal.

b. The appendix testis is attached to the upper pole of the testis and may undergo torsion, causing acute testicular pain.

c. The tunica albuginea lies around the testis and is covered superficially by the tunica vaginalis, the remnant of the foetal processus vaginalis.

e. The dartos muscle is directly subcutaneous in the scrotum. The three layers of spermatic fascia, including the cremasteric, lie directly deep to dartos.

5.16

d. Erection is controlled by the parasympathetic nervous system. The sympathetic system stimulates ejaculation.

Explanations

a. The tunica albuginea of the penis, which is not continuous with that of the testis, ensheathes the corpora cavernosa, allowing straight expansion of these structures during erection.

b. The penile urethra runs within the corpus spongiosum, which expands to form the glans penis.

c. The penis is supplied by three pairs of arteries: the artery of the bulb, the dorsal artery of the penis and the deep artery of the penis.

e. Bulbospongiosus arises from the perineal body and inserts into the perineal membrane and clasps the base of the corpus spongiosum. Its contraction therefore expels the terminal drips of urine from the penis.

5.17

d. The fallopian tubes contain an inner circular and outer longitudinal coat of smooth muscle, which assist in the progress of the ovum to the uterus following ovulation.

Explanations

a. The fundus lies superior to the entrance of the fallopian tubes into the uterus. It is the most superior part of the uterus and is palpable during bimanual vaginal examination or pregnancy.

b. The cornu of the uterus is the point at which the fundus joins the body and is also the point of entry of the uterine tubes into the uterus.

c. The infundibulum of the fallopian tubes bare fimbrae. They are the trumpet-shaped expansions at their distal end. The ampulla is the wider part of the tube, which arises from the isthmus.

e. The upper part of the uterus, including the fundus and uterine tubes, drains its lymph to the para-aortic lymph nodes. The lower part of the body drains into the internal and external iliac nodes.

5.18

b. The uterine artery ascends the lateral wall of the uterus, at the bottom of which it gives uterine and cervical branches. It ends by anastomosing with the ovarian artery along the fallopian tube.

Explanations

a. The normal position of the uterus is anteverted and anteflexed. The uterus is retroverted in 20% of females, rendering it impalpable on vaginal examination.

c. The cervix is attached to the posterior wall of the bladder by dense connective tissue. This is important in the spread of carcinoma of the cervix.

d. The uterus is formed by midline fusion of paramesonephric ducts.

e. The cardinal ligament is a thickening of the base of the broad ligament and passes from the cervix and lateral vaginal fornix to the lateral pelvic wall. It is traversed by the ureter, uterine artery and the inferior hypogastric plexus.

5.19

c. The suspensory ligament is attached to the fascia over psoas major.

Explanations

a. The ovarian vessels are contained within the suspensory ligament of the ovary, which connects the fascia overlying psoas major to the ovary.

b. On the right the ovarian vein drains into the inferior vena cava. This is a similar arrangement to the venous drainage of the testicles.

d. The lymphatics of the ovary pass with the blood vessels to drain into the para-aortic nodes.

e. The ovary is attached to the posterior aspect of the broad ligament.

5.20

a. The suspensory ligament of the ovary passes from the fascia over psoas major to attach to the ovary. The ovary lies on the posterior border of the broad ligament, a fold of peritoneum overlying the uterus and fallopian tubes.

Explanations

b. The round ligament is attached to the lateral angle of the uterus and runs in the anterior layer of the broad ligament. It passes through the inguinal ring to be attached the labium majus.

c. The uterine vessels enter the lateral wall of the uterus by running in the inferior free border of the broad ligament.

d. The fallopian tube runs in the superior border of the broad ligament.

e. The ovarian ligament runs in the broad ligament and attaches the ovary to the cornu of the uterus.

5.21

c. The ureter lies approximately 12 mm lateral to the supravaginal cervix. This accounts for the occurrence of hydronephrosis as a complication of disseminated carcinoma of the cervix.

Explanations

a. The anterior part of the cervix is in contact with the bladder and supravaginal cervix. The posterior part is covered by the peritoneum of the pouch of Douglas.

b. The vagina is related anteriorly to the base of the bladder and the urethra. The upper part of the posterior wall of the vagina is covered by the peritoneum of the pouch of Douglas.

d. The lower vagina is supplied by the perineal and posterior labial branches of the pudendal nerve. The upper part is sensitive only to stretch, with afferent fibres running with sympathetic nerves.

e. The lymph from the lower 1/3 of the vagina drains into the superficial inguinal nodes. The upper 2/3 drain into the internal and external iliac nodes.

5.22

a. The common iliac artery divides into its internal and external branches over the sacroiliac joint.

Explanations

b. The internal iliac artery divides into anterior and posterior branches. The external iliac artery passes under the inguinal ligament to become the femoral artery.

c. The ovarian artery is a branch of the aorta. Like the testis, the ovary descends during foetal life, dragging its blood supply and lymph drainage with it.

d. The inferior epigastric artery is a branch of the external iliac artery, just before it passes below the inguinal ligament. The inferior epigastric vessels are an important landmark in hernia surgery, as a direct inguinal hernia will emerge medial, and an indirect hernia lateral, to them.

e. The obturator artery is a branch of the internal iliac artery, it passes through the obturator foramen with the obturator nerve and vein to enter the medial compartment of the thigh.

5.23

d. Pubovaginalis slings around the vagina posteriorly, having arisen from the symphysis pubis. It contracts at the end of micturition to assist the urethral sphincter in terminating the stream of urine.

Explanations

a. Contraction of the bladder is initiated via parasympathetic fibres running in the pelvic splanchnic nerves.

b. The sphincter urethrae, or external urethral sphincter, is innervated by the perineal branch of the pudendal nerve.

c. The internal urethral sphincter acts principally to prevent retrograde ejaculation. It is, therefore, innervated by sympathetic fibres.

e. A lumbar cord transection results in an unopposed reflex arc not inhibited by higher centres. Bladder fullness, therefore, leads to spontaneous initiation of micturition.

5.24

d. The perineal branch is sensory to the skin of the scrotum and the labium majus.

Explanations

a. The pudendal nerve exits the pelvis through the greater sciatic foramen and re-enters through the lesser sciatic foramen to run along the lateral wall of the pelvis.

b. This is Alcock's canal, which contains the pudendal nerve and vessels.

c. The dorsal branch is sensory to the penis/clitoris.

e. The perineal branch of the pudendal nerve gives branches to the muscles of the urogenital diaphragm.

6

Head and Neck

QUESTIONS

6.1 Which statement about the neurocranium is correct?
- [ ] **a.** The bregma is the adult remnant of the posterior fontanelle.
- [ ] **b.** The metopic suture usually disappears in the first year of life.
- [ ] **c.** The anterior fontanelle is not palpable past 1 year of age.
- [ ] **d.** Six bones make up the adult neurocranium.
- [ ] **e.** The pterion represents the thinnest part of the lateral skull.

6.2 Which statement regarding the foramina of the skull is correct?
- [ ] **a.** The inferior ophthalmic vein passes through the inferior orbital fissure.
- [ ] **b.** The foramen spinosum connects the middle cranial fossa with the infratemporal fossa.
- [ ] **c.** The foramen ovale transmits the maxillary division of the trigeminal nerve.
- [ ] **d.** The optic nerve enters the skull in the anterior cranial fossa.
- [ ] **e.** The hypoglossal nerve exits the skull via the jugular foramen.

6.3 Which statement best describes the cranial fossae?
- ☐ **a.** The middle cranial fossa contains the cribriform plate.
- ☐ **b.** The anterior cranial fossa contains the pituitary gland.
- ☐ **c.** The middle cranial fossa is floored by the sphenoid and temporal bones.
- ☐ **d.** The internal acoustic meatus lies in the middle cranial fossa.
- ☐ **e.** The occipital lobe lies in the posterior cranial fossa.

6.4 Which statement concerning the development of the face is *incorrect*?
- ☐ **a.** Frontonasal process forms the nose.
- ☐ **b.** Frontonasal process forms the premaxilla.
- ☐ **c.** Maxillary processes fuse in the midline.
- ☐ **d.** Maxillary processes forms the entire palate.
- ☐ **e.** Mandibular processes fuse in the midline.

6.5 Which statement best describes the branchial arches and their derivatives?
- ☐ **a.** Five branchial arches form in human embryos.
- ☐ **b.** The ossicles of the middle ear are all skeletal derivatives of the first arch.
- ☐ **c.** The muscles of facial expression are derived from the second arch.
- ☐ **d.** The nerve of the third arch is the vagus.
- ☐ **e.** The artery of the first arch forms part of the internal carotid artery.

6.6 Which of the following statements about the eye are *incorrect*?

   ☐ **a.** Aqueous humour is drained via the canal of Schlemm.

   ☐ **b.** Greatest visual acuity is found at the macula densa.

   ☐ **c.** The optic nerve is invested by all three meningeal layers.

   ☐ **d.** The central artery of the retina is an end artery.

   ☐ **e.** Parasympathetic fibres from the oculomotor nerve innervate the lacrimal gland.

6.7 Which statement best describes the muscles of the eye?

   ☐ **a.** The superior and inferior obliques arise from the tendinous ring.

   ☐ **b.** The superior oblique is innervated by the oculomotor nerve.

   ☐ **c.** Sphincter pupillae is innervated by sympathetic nerves.

   ☐ **d.** Oculomotor nerve paralysis causes a complete ptosis.

   ☐ **e.** Closure of the eye is controlled by the facial nerve.

6.8 Which statement best describes the middle ear?

   ☐ **a.** The medial wall is formed by the tympanic membrane.

   ☐ **b.** The epitympanic recess contains the incus and head of the stapes.

   ☐ **c.** The internal jugular vein is related to its roof.

   ☐ **d.** It communicates with the mastoid air cells inferiorly.

   ☐ **e.** The Eustachian tube runs from the anterior wall of the middle ear to the oropharynx.

6.9 Which statement about the nasal septum is correct?
- ☐ **a.** Is formed by the septal cartilage posteriorly.
- ☐ **b.** Is formed by the perpendicular plate of the ethmoid postero-inferiorly.
- ☐ **c.** Is lined by mucoperiosteum throughout.
- ☐ **d.** Little's area overlies the vomer.
- ☐ **e.** The sphenopalatine artery courses over the septum.

6.10 Consider the lateral wall of the nasal cavity, which statement describes it the best?
- ☐ **a.** It is formed principally by the ethmoid bone.
- ☐ **b.** The nasal bone forms the anterior part of the lateral wall.
- ☐ **c.** The inferior concha is part of the maxilla.
- ☐ **d.** The superior concha is part of the maxilla.
- ☐ **e.** The superior meatus lies above the superior turbinate.

6.11 Which statement about the maxillary sinus is *incorrect*?
- ☐ **a.** Is lined by respiratory mucous membrane.
- ☐ **b.** Forms the floor of the orbit via its roof.
- ☐ **c.** Is drained from its most dependent part.
- ☐ **d.** Drains into the middle meatus.
- ☐ **e.** Is supplied by branches of the maxillary nerve.

6.12 Which statement describing the ethmoid sinuses is *not* correct?
- ☐ **a.** They lie between the orbit and the nasal cavity.
- ☐ **b.** They form six distinct cavities.
- ☐ **c.** The anterior ethmoidal air cells drain into the middle meatus.
- ☐ **d.** The posterior ethmoidal air cells drain into the superior meatus.
- ☐ **e.** Are supplied by branches from both the ophthalmic and maxillary branches of the trigeminal nerve.

6.13 Which statement concerning the paranasal sinuses is *not* correct?

☐ **a.** The sphenoid sinuses are medial to the cavernous sinus.

☐ **b.** The sphenoid sinuses open into the nasal cavity behind the superior concha.

☐ **c.** The frontal sinuses are not present at birth.

☐ **d.** The frontal sinus is related to the orbit.

☐ **e.** The frontal sinus drains into the superior meatus.

6.14 Which of the following statements does *not* correctly describe the oral cavity?

☐ **a.** Taste sensation for the posterior 1/3 of the tongue is supplied by the glossopharyngeal nerve.

☐ **b.** The sensory innervation for the anterior 2/3 of the tongue is provided by the trigeminal nerve.

☐ **c.** The four extrinsic muscles of the tongue are supplied by the hypoglossal nerve.

☐ **d.** Lesions of the hypoglossal nerve cause ipsilateral deviation of the tongue on protrusion.

☐ **e.** The teeth are innervated by divisions of the trigeminal nerve.

6.15 Which statement best describes the anatomy of the tongue?

☐ **a.** The anterior 1/3 is separated from the posterior 2/3 by the sulcus terminalis.

☐ **b.** Receives its blood supply from a direct branch of the external carotid artery.

☐ **c.** The posterior 1/3 drains lymph to the lower part of the deep cervical chain of lymph nodes.

☐ **d.** Common sensation to the anterior 2/3 of the tongue is derived from the facial nerve.

☐ **e.** The intrinsic muscles of the tongue are all innervated by the facial nerve.

6.16 Which of the following is *not* true of the palatine tonsil?

☐ **a.** Has the palatopharyngeal arch as a direct anterior relation.

☐ **b.** Is separated by its capsule from the superior constrictor of the pharynx.

☐ **c.** Derives its blood supply principally from the facial artery.

☐ **d.** Has the paratonsillar vein as a lateral relation.

☐ **e.** Drains its lymph to nodes along the internal jugular vein.

6.17 Which statement *incorrectly* describes the muscles of mastication?

☐ **a.** Dislocation of the temporomandibular joint usually occurs anteriorly.

☐ **b.** The medial pterygoid takes origin from the lateral pterygoid plate.

☐ **c.** Of the muscles of mastication only the lateral pterygoid is involved in protracting the mandible.

☐ **d.** All the muscles of mastication are innervated by the maxillary division of the trigeminal nerve.

☐ **e.** All of the muscles of mastication are supplied by branches of the maxillary artery.

6.18 Which statement regarding the parotid gland is correct?

☐ **a.** The parotid duct opens into the oral cavity opposite the second lower molar tooth.

☐ **b.** The parotid duct runs deep to masseter throughout its course.

☐ **c.** Preganglionic parasympathetic fibres innervating the parotid originate in the superior salivary nucleus.

☐ **d.** Postganglionic parasympathetic fibres originate in the submandibular ganglion.

☐ **e.** Sympathetic innervation to the parotid follows the external carotid artery.

6.19 Which of the following statements best describes the salivary glands?

- ☐ **a.** The stylomandibular ligament separates the submandibular and sublingual glands.
- ☐ **b.** The parotid duct is also known as Wharton's duct.
- ☐ **c.** Stensen's duct empties alongside the frenulum of the tongue.
- ☐ **d.** Postganglionic parasympathetic fibres to the submandibular gland are transmitted via the chorda tympani nerve.
- ☐ **e.** The submandibular gland is related to the posterior border of mylohyoid.

6.20 Which statement about the surface anatomy of the neck is true?

- ☐ **a.** The hard palate lies at the same level as the atlas.
- ☐ **b.** The hyoid lies at the level of C4.
- ☐ **c.** The cricoid lies at the level of C5.
- ☐ **d.** The oesophagus commences at the level of C7.
- ☐ **e.** The carotid tubercle lies at the level of C3.

6.21 Which of the following statements about the anterior triangle of the neck is *incorrect*?

- ☐ **a.** Lies between the midline, the mandible and the anterior border of sternocleidomastoid.
- ☐ **b.** Is further divided by the digastric and omohyoid muscles.
- ☐ **c.** Contains the submandibular gland.
- ☐ **d.** Contains the external jugular vein.
- ☐ **e.** Contains the carotid sheath.

6.22 Which of these statements about the posterior triangle of the neck is *incorrect?*

- [ ] **a.** It is bounded by the sternocleidomastoid, trapezius and the middle third of the clavicle.
- [ ] **b.** It contains the spinal accessory nerve.
- [ ] **c.** The spinal accessory nerve can be identified at the posterior border of sternocleidomastoid.
- [ ] **d.** It is floored by prevertebral fascia.
- [ ] **e.** It contains the first part of the subclavian artery.

6.23 Which statement about the fascial planes of the neck is *not* correct?

- [ ] **a.** The investing layer of fascia completely surrounds the neck.
- [ ] **b.** The investing layer of fascia contributes to the capsule of the parotid gland.
- [ ] **c.** The prevertebral fascia is continuous with the axillary sheath.
- [ ] **d.** The pretracheal fascia has two layers.
- [ ] **e.** The prevertebral fascia merges with the pericardium.

6.24 Which statement concerning the muscles of the neck is true?

- [ ] **a.** The tendon of omohyoid overlies the internal jugular vein.
- [ ] **b.** The suprahyoid muscles are supplied by the ansa cervicalis.
- [ ] **c.** Sternothyroid lies superficial to sternohyoid.
- [ ] **d.** Stylohyoid is supplied by the glossopharyngeal nerve.
- [ ] **e.** Mylohyoid is supplied by the facial nerve.

6.25 Which of the following statements describing the pharynx is *incorrect*?

- ☐ **a.** The nasopharynx derives its sensory innervation from the trigeminal nerve.
- ☐ **b.** The glossopharyngeal nerve passes between the superior and middle constrictors.
- ☐ **c.** It is lined by stratified squamous epithelium throughout.
- ☐ **d.** The weakest part of the muscular wall is at the level of the inferior constrictor.
- ☐ **e.** It ends at the level of C6.

6.26 Which of the following statements about the larynx is *incorrect*?

- ☐ **a.** The laryngeal inlet opens into the laryngopharynx.
- ☐ **b.** The vestibule of the larynx lies between the vestibular fold and the vocal fold.
- ☐ **c.** The narrowest part of the larynx in an adult is at the level of the vocal folds.
- ☐ **d.** The cricothyroid membrane forms the vocal ligament.
- ☐ **e.** The infraglottic portion is supplied by the inferior thyroid artery.

6.27 Which statement, concerning the larynx is correct?

- ☐ **a.** The supraglottic part of the larynx drains to the upper deep cervical nodes.
- ☐ **b.** The vocal folds drain to the inferior deep cervical nodes.
- ☐ **c.** The cricothyroid is the only muscle to abduct the vocal cords.
- ☐ **d.** The posterior cricoarytenoid is supplied by the superior laryngeal nerve.
- ☐ **e.** The vocal folds are cushioned by a layer of submucosa.

6.28 Which statement about the blood supply of the thyroid is correct?

☐ **a.** Inferior thyroid artery is a branch of the external carotid artery.

☐ **b.** Inferior thyroid artery normally supplies the superior and inferior parathyroids.

☐ **c.** Thyroidea ima usually arises from the arch of the aorta.

☐ **d.** Middle thyroid vein drains into the brachiocephalic vein.

☐ **e.** External laryngeal nerve is closely related to the inferior thyroid vessels.

6.29 Which statement regarding the development of the thyroid and parathyroids is *not* correct?

☐ **a.** The thyroid is in its approximate adult position at birth.

☐ **b.** The foramen caecum is an embryological remnant of the thyroid's development.

☐ **c.** Levator glandulae thyroidae is an embryological remnant of the thyroid's development.

☐ **d.** The inferior parathyroid glands develop from the 3rd branchial arch.

☐ **e.** The superior parathyroids are more variable in position than the inferior parathyroids.

6.30 Which statement concerning the parathyroid glands is correct?

☐ **a.** Four glands are present in 50% of subjects.

☐ **b.** The superior parathyroid lies above the superior thyroid artery.

☐ **c.** The parathyroids have a combined weight of 1g.

☐ **d.** Oxyphil cells secrete parathyroid hormone.

☐ **e.** The superior parathyroid lies within the pretracheal fascia.

6.31 Which statement best describes the external carotid artery and its branches?

☐ **a.** The anterior part of the scalp is supplied by the facial branch of the external carotid.

☐ **b.** The maxillary artery is divided into three parts by the lateral pterygoid muscle.

☐ **c.** The facial artery is easily palpable at the anterior border of masseter.

☐ **d.** The lingual artery gives the superior laryngeal artery as a branch.

☐ **e.** The middle meningeal artery is a branch of the facial artery.

6.32 Which statement regarding the lymphatic drainage of the head and neck is *incorrect*?

☐ **a.** All the lymph drainage from the face enters the deep cervical nodes.

☐ **b.** The left deep cervical nodes drain into the thoracic duct.

☐ **c.** The right lymphatic duct drains into the junction between the right internal jugular and brachiocephalic veins.

☐ **d.** The superficial cervical nodes lie along the external jugular vein.

☐ **e.** The jugulo-omohyoid node is easily palpable when enlarged.

ANSWERS

6.1

e. The pterion represents the remnant of the sphenoidal fontanelle in adults, and is the thinnest part of the skull. The middle meningeal artery lies deep to the pterion and is particularly vulnerable to damage following blows to this region.

Explanations

a. The bregma is the adult remnant of the anterior fontanelle. It is formed by the intersection of the sagittal and coronal sutures. The lambda (or asterion) is the adult remnant of the posterior fontanelle, and is formed by the intersection of the lambdoid and sagittal sutures.

b. The frontal bone is separated into two parts by the metopic suture at birth. Fusion usually starts in the second year of life and is complete by age 7 years. This suture may persist, however, into adult life, occurring in up to 7.4% of the population. This suture should not be mistaken for a fracture line.

c. The anterior fontanelle is palpable until approximately 18 months of age. The posterior fontanelle is not usually palpable past the first year.

d. Eight bones make up the adult neurocranium. There are two paired sets: the parietal and temporal bones; and four individual bones: the frontal, occipital, sphenoid and ethmoid bones.

6.2

b. This is also true of the foramen ovale. The middle meningeal artery enters the skull via the foramen spinosum.

Explanations

a. Both the superior and inferior ophthalmic veins pass through the superior orbital fissure, along with the oculomotor, trochlear and abducent nerves, as well as the ophthalmic division of the trigeminal nerve.

c. The maxillary division is transmitted through the foramen rotundum to enter the pterygopalatine fossa. The foramen ovale transmits the mandibular division to the infratemporal fossa as well as the lesser petrosal branch of the glossopharyngeal nerve.

d. The optic nerve enters the skull through the optic canal into the middle cranial fossa.

e. The hypoglossal nerve exits the skull through the hypoglossal canal.

6.3

c. The floor of the middle cranial fossa is made up of the body and greater wing of the sphenoid as well as the squamous temporal bone. The middle cranial fossa contains many foramina and canals, and is therefore vulnerable to fracture.

Explanations

a. The cribriform plate forms part of the floor of the anterior cranial fossa along with the orbital plate of the frontal bone and the lesser wings of the sphenoid. A fracture of the cribriform plate may lead to leakage of cerebrospinal fluid through the nose (cerebrospinal fluid rhinorrhoea).

b. The pituitary gland lies in the hypophyseal fossa, above the body of the sphenoid bone, which is in the middle cranial fossa.

d. The internal acoustic meatus lies in the posterior cranial fossa, with the VIIth and VIIIth cranial nerves entering after leaving the brainstem. The border of the middle cranial fossa is the petrous temporal bone, to which is attached the tentorium cerebelli.

e. The occipital lobe lies in the middle cranial fossa. The posterior cranial fossa is the space inferior to the tentorium cerebelli and contains the cerebellum and brainstem.

6.4

d. The palate is derived from the maxillary processes with the exception of the anterior portion formed by the premaxilla.

Explanations

a. The frontonasal process projects from the primitive cranium and forms the nose, nasal septum, nostril and philtrum of the upper lip.

b. The premaxilla is the anterior portion of the upper jaw.

c. The two maxillary processes fuse with the frontonasal process slightly lateral to the midline. However, the hard palate is formed by midline fusion of the two maxillary processes. Failure of this fusion leads to cleft lip and palate.

e. The mandibular processes fuse in the midline and form the lower jaw. Failure of this fusion leads to the rare condition of cleft lower lip.

6.5

c. The muscles of facial expression, stapedius, stylohyoid and the posterior belly of digastric are all derived from the second arch. All these muscles, therefore, share a common innervation by the second arch nerve (the facial nerve).

Explanations

a. The branchial arches form as six mesodermal condensations in the lateral primitive pharynx and grow forwards to fuse in the midline. The fifth arch is rudimentary and does not persist. Skeletal and muscular components are derived from each arch, with each arch having its own nerve and artery.

b. The incus and malleus are derived from the first arch. The stapes is derived from the second arch along with the styloid process, stylohyoid ligament and the lesser horn and superior part of the body of the hyoid bone.

d. The vagus provides innervation for the fourth and sixth arches via its superior and inferior laryngeal branches. The nerves for the first, second and third arches are the mandibular, facial and glossopharyngeal, respectively.

e. The artery for the first arch contributes to the maxillary artery. The third arch artery gives rise to the common and internal carotids on each side.

6.6

e. The lacrimal gland is innervated by parasympathetic fibres travelling in the facial nerve, transmitted to the orbit via the maxillary division of the trigeminal nerve.

Explanations

a. Aqueous humour is produced by the ciliary body in the posterior chamber. It enters the anterior chamber through the pupil and then is drained via the canal of Schlemm. Obstruction of this canal can lead to glaucoma.

b. Visual acuity is at its greatest on the portion of the retina called the macula.

c. This allows raised cerebrospinal fluid pressure to be transmitted via the subarachnoid space to the orbit, which may compress venous drainage of the eye. The consequent swelling of the optic disc (papilloedema) can be detected by ophthalmoscopy.

d. The central artery of the retina is a branch of the ophthalmic artery and pierces the optic disc to supply the retina. The retina has no collateral circulation, therefore occlusion causes instant blindness.

6.7

e. Orbicularis oculi shuts the eyes when contracted. It is a muscle of facial expression and is, therefore, innervated by the facial nerve.

Explanations

a. The four rectus muscles arise from the tendinous ring around the optic foramen, and medial part of the superior orbital fissure. Superior oblique arises superior and medial to the ring and inferior oblique arises from the floor of the orbit.

b. All the extra-ocular muscles are innervated by the oculomotor nerve except the superior oblique and the lateral rectus, which are innervated by the trochlear nerve and the abducent nerve, respectively.

c. Sphincter pupillae is innervated by parasympathetic fibres from the oculomotor nerve. These fibres are carried by the short ciliary nerves. Dilator pupillae is innervated by sympathetic fibres carried via the long ciliary nerves.

d. Levator palpebrae superioris is responsible for elevating the upper eyelid and is innervated by the oculomotor nerve. It does, however, have some smooth muscle fibres in its deep part supplied by sympathetic fibres. Oculomotor nerve paralysis, therefore, causes a marked ptosis with some sparing of function due to sympathetic supply.

6.8

b. The epitympanic recess is the part of the tympanic cavity above the tympanic membrane. It contains the incus and head of the stapes, and provides a space for the growth of middle ear masses (e.g. cholesteatoma).

Explanations

a. The lateral wall of the tympanic cavity (or middle ear) is formed by the tympanic membrane and the tympanic ring. The medial wall separates the middle ear from the internal ear and contains the round window (fenestra cochleae) and oval window (fenestra vestibule). The oval window is attached to the stapes.

c. The bulb of the internal jugular vein lies below the floor of the middle ear. The middle cranial fossa lies above the roof, separated by the tegmen tympani, a thin plate of the temporal bone.

d. The middle ear communicates with the mastoid air cells via the mastoid antrum, which opens into the epitympanic recess.

e. The Eustachian tube connects the anterior wall of the middle ear to the lateral wall of the nasopharynx. It opens close to an accumulation of lymphoid tissue which may block the tube when inflamed. This may lead to recurrent otitis media with effusion (glue ear).

6.9

e. The sphenopalatine artery is a terminal branch of the maxillary artery and courses over the nasal septum. The sphenopalatine artery ramifies over the conchae and meatuses.

Explanations

a. The septal cartilage represents the unossified part of the ethmoid bone and lies anteriorly. The septum is often deviated.

b. The perpendicular plate of the ethmoid forms the postero-superior part of the nasal septum. The vomer forms the postero-inferior part.

c. The septum is lined by mucoperiosteum (overlying the bony parts) and mucoperochondrium (overlying the cartilage). Although these layers are closely adherent to the septum they can be stripped off, for example, in septoplasty.

d. Little's area is the point of anastomosis of the sphenopalatine artery, the ascending branch of the greater palatine artery and the septal branch of the superior labial artery. It is a common sight for epistaxis. As it overlies the lower anterior part of the septum it is easily accessible for cautery.

6.10

b. The nasal bones form part of the anterosuperior part of the lateral wall of the nose.

Explanations

a. The majority of the lateral wall of the nose is made up by the maxilla. A large defect in the medial aspect of the maxilla is closed by parts of the ethmoid, palatine, inferior conchae and sphenoid bones.

c. The inferior concha (or turbinate) is a bone in itself, it articulates with the maxilla and the palatine bone.

d. The superior and middle conchae (or turbinates) are part of the lateral mass of the ethmoid.

e. The superior meatus lies below the superior concha (or turbinate).

6.11

c. The maxillary sinus is drained from its least dependent part, near the top. It is therefore prone to sinusitis as it drains poorly.

Explanations

a. All the nasal sinuses are lined by respiratory mucous membrane.

b. The walls of the maxillary sinus are shaped like an inverted triangle, the base of which lies superiorly and forms the floor of the orbit. The orbit is therefore subject to invasion from a carcinoma of the maxillary sinus. The orbital process of the palatine bone also forms a small part of the orbit posteriorly.

d. The maxillary sinus drains into the middle meatus.

e. The infraorbital and superior alveolar branches of the maxillary nerve supply the maxillary sinus. The superior alveolar nerves also supply the upper teeth. The close relationship of the maxillary sinus to the upper teeth means that it is prone to infection from dental caries and broken roots after unsuccessful extractions of upper teeth.

6.12

b. The ethmoid sinuses are divided into numerous air cells by bony septa. These are usually grouped into anterior middle and posterior air cells for the purposes of description, but there may be as many as 18 cells on each side.

Explanations

a. The ethmoidal sinuses lie between the nose and the orbit. Infection from the ethmoid sinuses may therefore invade the orbit, causing orbital cellulitis.

c. This is correct.

d. The posterior air cells do drain into the superior meatus, the middle air cells drain into the middle meatus. One of the middle air cells projects into the middle meatus forming the ethmoidal bulla.

e. The ethmoid sinuses are supplied by branches from both these branches of the trigeminal nerve. Thus pain from the ethmoid sinuses may be referred to the territory of either branch.

6.13

e. The frontal sinus drains into the middle meatus.

Explanations

a. The sphenoid sinuses lie in the body of the sphenoid bone. They are related superiorly to the pituitary fossa and middle cranial fossa, and laterally to the cavernous sinus and internal carotid artery.

b. The sphenoid sinuses open into the spheno-ethmoidal recess which lies behind the superior concha.

c. The frontal sinuses start to develop in the second year of life. They are the only paranasal sinuses not present at birth.

d. The frontal sinus is related to the orbit and to the anterior cranial fossa. Infection of the frontal sinus may therefore lead to the formation of a frontal lobe abscess.

6.14

c. The four extrinsic muscles of the tongue are: genioglossus, hyoglossus, styloglossus and palatoglossus. All the intrinsic and extrinsic muscles are innervated by the hypoglossal nerve apart from palatoglossus which is supplied by the vagus.

Explanations

a. The glossopharyngeal nerve contains sensory fibres, including taste, from the posterior third of the tongue and oropharynx.

b. Somatic sensory innervation for the anterior 2/3 of the tongue is provided by the lingual nerve, a branch of the mandibular division of the trigeminal nerve. Taste fibres from this area are conveyed by the chorda tympani, a branch of the facial nerve.

d. Damage to the hypoglossal nerve results in an ipsilateral paralysis and consequent wasting of tongue muscles. On protrusion of the tongue deviation will be towards the affected side. The palsy of the tongue is complete because although palatoglossus is supplied by the vagus nerve, it plays no part in tongue movement.

e. The teeth are innervated by divisions of the trigeminal nerve.

6.15

b. The tongue is supplied by the lingual branch of the external carotid artery.

Explanations

a. The sulcus terminalis separates the anterior 2/3 of the tongue, bearing papillae, from the posterior 1/3 which bears lymphoid nodules. These nodules complete the ring of lymphoid tissue made up by the adenoids and palatine tonsils (Waldeyer's ring).

c. The posterior 1/3 of the tongue drains to the upper part of the deep cervical chain. The anterior 2/3 drains into the lower part via the submental and submandibular nodes. The tip of the tongue drains into the submental nodes.

d. The chorda tympani, a branch of the facial nerve, supplies taste fibres to the anterior 2/3 of the tongue. Common sensation is supplied by the mandibular division of the trigeminal nerve via its lingual branch.

e. The intrinsic muscles of the tongue are all supplied by the hypoglossal nerve.

6.16

a. The palatoglossal arch, containing the palatoglossus muscle, lies directly anterior to the tonsil. The palatopharyngeal arch, containing the palatopharyngeus muscle, lies directly behind it.

Explanations

b. The tonsillar fossa is floored by the superior constrictor. The tonsillar capsule separates the tonsil from this muscle and is the plane of dissection to be sought in tonsillectomy.

c. The tonsil derives its major blood supply from the tonsillar branch of the facial artery. It also has a blood supply from the lingual, ascending palatine and ascending pharyngeal arteries. The rich blood supply explains the severity of bleeding that can occur from the tonsillar bed following tonsillectomy.

d. The palatine tonsil drains to the paratonsillar vein, which lies just lateral to the tonsillar capsule. If it is damaged during tonsillectomy it causes bleeding.

e. The lymph from the tonsil drains through vessels which pierce the superior constrictor of the pharynx and empties into lymph nodes along the internal jugular vein.

6.17

d. The muscles of mastication are all innervated by the mandibular division of the trigeminal nerve.

Explanations

a. The temporomandibular joint is mobile anteriorly and slides forwards, out of the mandibular fossa, when the mouth is opened.

b. The medial pterygoid takes origin via a larger deep head from the medial surface of the lateral pterygoid plate and a superficial head from the tuberosity of the maxilla and pyramidal process of the palatine bone. The lateral pterygoid also has two heads: the inferior head takes origin from the lateral surface of the lateral pterygoid plate and the superior from the roof of the infratemporal fossa.

c. The other muscles of mastication namely temporalis, masseter and the medial pterygoid all act to elevate the mandible. Retraction is achieved by the posterior fibres of temporalis.

e. The muscles of mastication are all supplied by branches of the maxillary artery, a terminal branch of the external carotid artery.

6.18

e. The sympathetic supply to the head and neck is conveyed by the arterial supply.

Explanations

a. The parotid duct is also known as Stensen's duct and opens into the oral cavity opposite the second upper molar tooth.

b. The parotid duct emerges from the anterior border of the gland to run anteriorly, superficial to masseter, before turning medially to pierce buccinator and enter the oral cavity.

c. Preganglionic parasympathetic fibres originate in the inferior salivary nucleus of the glossopharyngeal nerve follow the tympanic branch and then travel to the otic ganglion via the lesser petrosal nerve.

d. The submandibular ganglion is the origin for postganglionic parasympathetic fibres for the other salivary glands, which are conveyed by the lingual nerve. The otic ganglion is the origin for post-ganglionic fibres to the parotid, which are transmitted to the gland via the auriculotemporal nerve.

6.19

e. Each submandibular gland has a larger superficial part and a smaller deep part. The two are continuous posteriorly, and the anterior concavity is occupied by the posterior border of the mylohyoid muscle.

Explanations

a. The stylomandibular ligament separates the parotid and submandibular glands.

b. The parotid duct is also known as Stensen's duct. Wharton's duct is the name given to the submandibular duct.

c. Stensen's duct opens opposite the 2nd upper molar tooth. Whartonís duct empties alongside the frenulum of the tongue.

d. Pre-ganglionic parasympathetic fibres are carried via the chorda tympani nerve (branch of the facial nerve) to the submandibular ganglion. Post-ganglionic parasympathetic fibres are then conveyed via the lingual nerve to the sub-mandibular and sublingual glands.

6.20

a. The hard palate is at the level of the atlas, C1.

Explanations

b. The hyoid lies at the level of C3.

c. The cricoid lies at the level of C6, which is also the level at which the larynx joins the trachea.

d. The oesophagus commences at the level of C6, which is also the level at which the inferior thyroid artery and the middle thyroid vein enter the thyroid gland.

e. The carotid tubercle, the bony point against which the pulsation of the carotid artery can be felt, lies at the level of C6, which is also the level at which the superior belly of omohyoid crosses the carotid sheath and the level of the middle cervical ganglion.

6.21

d. The external jugular vein passes across the posterior triangle.

Explanations

a. The triangle is bounded by the midline, the inferior border of the mandible and the anterior border of sternocleidomastoid.

b. These muscles further divide the triangle into the digastric, muscular and carotid triangles.

c. The submandibular gland lies in the digastric triangle which is bounded by the two bellies of digastric and the inferior border of the mandible.

e. The carotid sheath, containing the common carotid artery, internal jugular vein and vagus nerve, runs in the anterior triangle.

6.22

e. The posterior triangle contains the second part of the sub-clavian artery which underlies scalenus anterior.

Explanations

a. The posterior triangle has these boundaries and is roofed by the investing layer of deep cervical fascia, which runs between trapezius and sternocleidomastoid.

b. The accessory nerve is a relatively superficial structure which lies deep and is adherent to the investing cervical fascia.

c. The accessory nerve enters the posterior triangle at the junction of the upper 1/3 and lower 2/3 of the posterior border of sternocleidomastoid.

d. The prevertebral fascia overlying the scalenes, levator scapulae and splenius capitis forms the floor of the posterior triangle.

6.23

e. The pretracheal fascia merges inferiorly with the pericardium.

Explanations

a. The investing layer of fascia arises from the ligamentum nuchae and surrounds the entire neck, splitting to enclose the sternocleidomastoid and trapezius muscles.

b. The investing layer contributes to the capsules of both the parotid and submandibular glands. It is attached above to the external occipital protuberance, mastoid process, zygomatic arch and the mandible.

c. The prevertebral fascial is continuous with the axillary sheath which encloses the subclavian artery and brachial plexus.

d. The anterior layer encloses the infrahyoid muscles and the posterior layer forms the fascial capsule of the thyroid gland.

6.24

a. The flattened tendon of omohyoid is bound to the clavicle by a fascial sling. It overlies the internal jugular vein, a useful landmark at operation.

Explanations

b. The ansa cervicalis supplies the infrahyoid muscles. It is made up of a superior root containing fibres from C1, which run with the hypoglossal nerve, and an inferior root which is composes of branches from C2 and C3.

c. Sternohyoid lies superior to sternothyroid. It is therefore the first of the strap muscles to be encountered during thyroidectomy.

d. Stylohyoid is supplied by the facial nerve. The three muscles arising from the styloid process are all supplied by a different cranial nerve. Stylopharyngeus is supplied by the glossopharyngeal nerve and styloglossus is supplied by the hypoglossal nerve.

e. Mylohyoid is supplied by the nerve to mylohyoid, a branch of the mandibular division of the trigeminal nerve.

6.25

c. The laryngopharynx is lined by columnar ciliated epithelium.

Explanations

a. The nasopharynx derives its sensory innervation from branches of the trigeminal nerve. The rest of the pharynx derives both its sensory and motor supply from the glosso-pharyngeal and vagus nerves.

b. The glossopharyngeal nerve passes between the superior and middle constrictors with the stylopharyngeus muscle, which it supplies.

d. The inferior constrictor has two parts, the cricopharyngeus and thyropharyngeus muscles. Between the two there is a gap (Killian's dehiscence), which is the weakest part of the muscle coat and the commonest site for herniation leading to the formation of a pharyngeal pouch.

e. The pharynx ends at the level of C6, where the laryn-gopharynx is continuous with the oesophagus.

6.26

b. The vestibule of the larynx lies between the laryngeal inlet and the vestibular fold. The ventricle lies between the vestibu-lar fold and the vocal fold.

Explanations

a. The laryngeal inlet is made up of the epiglottis anteriorly, the aryepiglottic folds laterally and the arytenoids and cor-niculate cartilages posteriorly.

c. The narrowest part of the larynx in an adult is the rima glottidis, the space between the vocal cords. The cricoid is the narrowest part of the airway of a child.

d. The vocal ligament, which forms the middle of the vocal cord, is formed by the thickened superior free border of the cricovocal membrane, which is the name given to the lateral cricothyroid ligament. The anterior (median) crico-thyroid ligament is the name given to the portion of the membrane between the thyroid and cricoid cartilages, and is an important site for the insertion of an emergency airway.

e. The supraglottic part of the larynx is supplied by the superior laryngeal artery, a branch of the external carotid. The infraglottic part is supplied by the inferior laryngeal artery, a branch of the inferior thyroid artery.

6.27

a. The area of the larynx above the vocal folds drains into the upper deep cervical nodes via nodes related to the thyrohyoid membrane.

Explanations

b. The vocal folds themselves are devoid of lymph drainage. The infraglottic part of the larynx drains into the lower deep cervical nodes. The vocal folds therefore represent a lymphatic watershed.

c. The only muscle to abduct the cords is the posterior cricoarytenoid. The cricothyroid tenses the vocal cords by approximating the thyroid cartilage to the cricoid cartilage.

d. The cricothyroid muscle is supplied by the superior laryngeal nerve; it is the only external muscle of the larynx. The posterior cricoarytenoid, along with all the other muscles of the larynx, is supplied by the recurrent laryngeal nerve.

e. The vocal folds have no submucosal layer, the mucosa is firmly attached to the vocal ligament. This accounts for the white appearance of the vocal folds and explains why laryngeal oedema does not involve the true vocal cords.

6.28

b. The superior and inferior parathyroid glands are usually supplied by the inferior thyroid artery. When these vessels are both tied in total thyroidectomy 30–40% of patients become hypocalcaemic due to parathyroid ischaemia.

Explanations

a. The inferior thyroid artery is a branch of the thyrocervical trunk which arises from the subclavian artery. The superior thyroid artery is a branch of the external carotid artery. The other branches of the thyrocervical trunk are the suprascapular and transverse cervical arteries.

c. The thyroidea ima, where present, usually arises from the brachiocephalic artery.

d. The middle thyroid vein drains into the internal jugular vein, which is therefore liable to damage at thyroidectomy resulting in severe bleeding.

e. The external laryngeal branch of the superior laryngeal nerve is related to this group of vessels and should be preserved during thyroidectomy to avoid voice change.

6.29

e. The inferior parathyroids are more variable in position than the superior. The thymus also develops from the 3rd branchial pouch, occasionally causing the inferior parathyroid to descend into the mediastinum.

Explanations

a. The thyroid is fully developed and in its adult position by the 6th month of intrauterine life.

b. The foramen caecum is the remnant of the start of the thyroid's development, which begins as a budding from the primitive pharynx. It is found at the junction between the anterior 2/3 and posterior 1/3 of the tongue.

c. The levator glandulae thyroidae is a fibrous cord which is the remnant of the descent of the thyroid from the primitive pharynx to the neck. A thyroglossal cyst or sinus may occur along this track.

d. The inferior parathyroid develops from the 3rd branchial pouch. The superior parathyroid, somewhat counter-intuitively, develops from the 4th branchial pouch.

6.30

e. The superior parathyroid lies within the pretracheal fascia, which forms the capsule of the thyroid gland. Its close relationship to the thyroid means that it is at risk during thyroidectomy. The inferior parathyroid usually also lies within this fascial capsule, although its position is more variable.

Explanations

a. There are four glands in 90% of subjects. The remainder have three, five or six. Therefore, an adenoma causing hypercalcaemia may lie in a fifth or a sixth gland.

b. The superior parathyroids lie on the posterior aspect of the gland above the inferior thyroid artery. The inferior para-thyroids lie below this artery and are related to the lower part of the thyroid lobe. The superior and inferior parathyroids are both supplied by the inferior thyroid artery.

c. A normal parathyroid weighs approximately 50 mg, so they have a combined weight of 200 mg.

d. Chief (or principal) cells secrete parathyroid hormone.

6.31

c. The facial artery runs over the submandibular gland, which it grooves deeply. It loops inferiorly, then upwards around the lower border of the mandible. It is easily palpable just anterior to the insertion of masseter.

Explanations

a. The anterior part of the scalp is predominantly supplied by the supraorbital and supratrochlear arteries, which are derived from the internal carotid via the ophthalmic artery.

b. The maxillary artery is divided into three parts by its relationship to the lateral pterygoid. The first part lies posterior to the muscle, the second part between its two heads and the third part anterior to it.

d. The superior laryngeal artery is a branch of the superior thyroid artery.

e. The middle meningeal artery is a branch of the first part of the maxillary artery. It passes vertically through the two rootlets of the auriculotemporal nerve to enter the middle cranial fossa through the foramen spinosum.

6.32

e. The jugulo-omohyoid node is closely related to the internal jugular vein and lies at the level of the tendon of omohyoid. At this point it is deep to sternocleidomastoid and is therefore not easily palpable. The jugulodigastric node (or tonsillar node), which lies behind the posterior body of the digastric, is easily palpable.

Explanations

a. The lymph drainage from the head and neck all eventually drains into the deep cervical nodes. The drainage from the face empties into deep cervical nodes via the submental, submandibular and pre-auricular nodes.

b. The deep cervical nodes coalesce to form the lymphatic trunk which drains into the thoracic duct on the left and the right lymphatic duct on the right.

c. The right lymphatic duct drains in a similar way to the thoracic duct, into the venous angle between the internal jugular and brachiocephalic veins.

d. The superficial cervical nodes lie along the external jugular vein. The anterior cervical nodes lie along the anterior jugular vein.

7

Central Nervous System and Spine

QUESTIONS

7.1 Which of the following statements about the cerebral hemispheres is correct?

- ☐ **a.** They occupy the anterior, middle and posterior cranial fossae.
- ☐ **b.** They are joined by the falx cerebri.
- ☐ **c.** Grey matter covers the entire surface of each hemisphere.
- ☐ **d.** The central sulcus separates them.
- ☐ **e.** The lateral sulcus separates the frontal and parietal lobes.

7.2 Which of the following statements regarding the cerebral cortex is true?

- ☐ **a.** The primary motor cortex lies in the frontal lobe.
- ☐ **b.** The primary somatosensory cortex lies in the frontal lobe.
- ☐ **c.** The primary auditory cortex lies in the parietal lobe.
- ☐ **d.** The primary visual cortex lies in the frontal lobe.
- ☐ **e.** Broca's speech area lies in the parietal lobe.

7.3 Which statement regarding the cerebellum is correct?
- □ **a.** The cerebellum occupies the posterior cranial fossa.
- □ **b.** It is attached to the pons by the superior cerebellar peduncle.
- □ **c.** It is divided into anterior and posterior lobes by the horizontal fissure.
- □ **d.** The cerebellar tonsil is found on its superior surface.
- □ **e.** It derives part of its blood supply from the circles of Willis.

7.4 Regarding the ventricular system and cerebrospinal fluid (CSF) production, which of the following statements is true?
- □ **a.** CSF is exclusively produced in the choroid plexi of the lateral ventricles.
- □ **b.** CSF passes from the 3rd to the 4th ventricle via the interventricular foramen.
- □ **c.** The 4th ventricle communicates directly with the subarachnoid space.
- □ **d.** The total daily production of CSF is approximately 150 ml.
- □ **e.** CSF is reabsorbed mainly through the arachnoid granulations in the inferior sagittal sinus.

7.5 Which statement about the meninges is most accurate?
- □ **a.** The dura mater has two distinct layers surrounding the brain and spinal cord.
- □ **b.** The major venous sinuses lie in the subdural space.
- □ **c.** Rupture of the middle meningeal artery causes a subarachnoid haemorrhage.
- □ **d.** Dura mater is thickened either side of the spinal cord to form the denticulate ligaments.
- □ **e.** The pia mater pierces the distal extreme of the dura as the filum terminale.

7.6 Which statement about the pituitary gland is correct?

☐ **a.** The posterior lobe is larger than the anterior lobe.

☐ **b.** The pituitary stalk connects the anterior lobe to the hypothalamus.

☐ **c.** It lies superior to the sphenoidal air sinuses.

☐ **d.** Both lobes develop as cerebral diverticulae.

☐ **e.** Pituitary tumours may cause a homonymous hemianopia.

7.7 Which of the following statements best describes the circle of Willis?

☐ **a.** It is formed by the terminal branches of the external carotid and basilar arteries.

☐ **b.** The ophthalmic artery is a branch of the circle.

☐ **c.** The middle cerebral artery forms part of the anterior circulation.

☐ **d.** The middle cerebral artery supplies the majority of the occipital lobe.

☐ **e.** The cerebellum is supplied by the circle.

7.8 Which statement is true of the venous drainage of the brain?

☐ **a.** The superior sagittal sinus usually empties into the left transverse sinus.

☐ **b.** The great cerebral vein empties into the inferior sagittal sinus.

☐ **c.** The inferior petrosal sinuses drain from the cavernous sinus into the sigmoid sinuses.

☐ **d.** The superior sagittal sinus is connected to the subarachnoid space.

☐ **e.** The superior cerebral veins drain into the cavernous sinus from above.

7.9 Which statement most accurately describes the olfactory nerve?

- ☐ **a.** The fibres of the olfactory cells run through the cribriform plate of the frontal bone.
- ☐ **b.** The nerve bundles are surrounded by all three meningeal layers.
- ☐ **c.** The olfactory tracts run on the medial surface of the respective hemispheres.
- ☐ **d.** Unilateral anosmia may commonly follow anterior cranial fossa fractures.
- ☐ **e.** The olfactory cortex is found in the parietal lobe.

7.10 Which statement about the optic nerve and tract is correct?

- ☐ **a.** The optic nerve is formed on the superficial surface of the retina.
- ☐ **b.** Fibres in the optic tract which subserve the nasal visual field cross in the optic chiasm.
- ☐ **c.** The majority of fibres in the optic tract pass to the brainstem.
- ☐ **d.** The optic radiation passes from the superior colliculus to the occipital cortex.
- ☐ **e.** The lower part of the retina is represented in the occipital cortex above the calcarine fissure.

7.11 Which of these statements about the oculomotor nerve is *not* correct?

- ☐ **a.** Its nuclei of origin are situated at the level of the inferior colliculus.
- ☐ **b.** It passes between the superior cerebellar and posterior cerebral arteries.
- ☐ **c.** It divides into a superior and inferior branch as it enters the orbit.
- ☐ **d.** Damage will result in a dilated pupil.
- ☐ **e.** Parasympathetic fibres are conveyed to the ciliary ganglion via the nerve to inferior rectus.

7.12 Which statement *does not* accurately describes the trochlear nerve?

- ☐ **a.** The nucleus is in the pons at the level of the inferior colliculus.
- ☐ **b.** Its nerve fibres decussate before the nerve leaves the brain.
- ☐ **c.** In emerges from posterior surface of the brainstem.
- ☐ **d.** It courses in the wall of the cavernous sinus.
- ☐ **e.** It enters the orbit by passing through the inferior orbital fissure.

7.13 Which statement about the maxillary nerve is *incorrect*?

- ☐ **a.** Is connected to the submandibular ganglion.
- ☐ **b.** Supplies the upper teeth.
- ☐ **c.** Contains sensory fibres for the hard palate.
- ☐ **d.** Contains sensory fibres for the soft palate.
- ☐ **e.** Its terminal branch passes through the inferior orbital fissure.

7.14 Which statement best describes the mandibular nerve?

- ☐ **a.** The anterior division supplies the four muscles of mastication.
- ☐ **b.** The auriculotemporal branch is medially related to the middle meningeal artery.
- ☐ **c.** Taste for the anterior 2/3rds of the tongue is conveyed by the lingual branch.
- ☐ **d.** The posterior division carries motor supply for the posterior belly of digastric.
- ☐ **e.** The inferior alveolar branch enters the mandible through the mental foramen.

7.15 Which statement best completes the following sentence? The abducent nerve:

- [ ] **a.** Runs in the wall of the cavernous sinus.
- [ ] **b.** Innervates the medial rectus.
- [ ] **c.** Passes through the tendinous ring.
- [ ] **d.** Emerges at the junction of the midbrain and the pons.
- [ ] **e.** If transected, leads to diplopia on looking to the contralateral side.

7.16 Which statement regarding the facial nerve is correct?

- [ ] **a.** The chorda tympani conveys parasympathetic fibres for the parotid gland.
- [ ] **b.** The main trunk of the facial nerve emerges from the stylomastoid foramen.
- [ ] **c.** It has five branches after exiting the skull.
- [ ] **d.** It lies deep to the retromandibular vein.
- [ ] **e.** In supranuclear palsy, weakness of the ipsilateral facial muscles would be noted.

7.17 Consider the vestibulocochlear nerve and its connections, which statement is *incorrect*?

- [ ] **a.** The vestibular portion of the nerve carries fibres subserving balance.
- [ ] **b.** It enters the brain at the cerebellopontine angle with the glossopharyngeal nerve.
- [ ] **c.** The auditory radiation passes from the medial geniculate body to the temporal lobe.
- [ ] **d.** The auditory cortex is bilaterally innervated.
- [ ] **e.** Efferent fibres from the vestibular nucleus pass to the cerebellum.

7.18 Which statement best completes the following sentence? The glossopharyngeal nerve:

☐ **a.** Gives preganglionic parasympathetic fibres to the submandibular ganglion.

☐ **b.** Contains no motor fibres.

☐ **c.** Supplies the aortic arch baroreceptors.

☐ **d.** Passes between the external carotid and the internal carotid arteries.

☐ **e.** Supplies common sensation to the posterior 2/3 of the tongue.

7.19 Which statement about the vagus nerve is *incorrect*?

☐ **a.** Runs in the carotid sheath superficial to the carotid artery and internal jugular vein.

☐ **b.** Passes anterior to the subclavian artery when entering the thorax.

☐ **c.** Gives sensory fibres to the tympanic membrane.

☐ **d.** Gives off the right recurrent laryngeal nerve in the root of the neck.

☐ **e.** Gives a motor supply to all the intrinsic muscles of the larynx.

7.20 Which statement about the accessory nerve is correct?

☐ **a.** The spinal root exits the skull through the foramen magnum.

☐ **b.** The spinal root is distributed via the vagus nerve.

☐ **c.** The spinal root contains fibres which supply sternocleidomastoid and trapezius.

☐ **d.** The cranial root pierces sternocleidomastoid.

☐ **e.** The cranial root passes across the posterior triangle of the neck.

7.21 Consider the spinal cord, which statement is most accurate?

- ☐ **a.** It tapers into the conus medullaris at the level of the 2nd sacral vertebra.
- ☐ **b.** It is supplied exclusively by the anterior and posterior spinal arteries.
- ☐ **c.** There are three symmetrical enlargements of the cord.
- ☐ **d.** The nerve roots emerging from the cord become progressively longer.
- ☐ **e.** The spinal nerve roots exit through the vertebral foramina.

7.22 Which statement about the spinal nerves is *incorrect*?

- ☐ **a.** There are 31 pairs.
- ☐ **b.** Their posterior root contains sensory afferent fibres.
- ☐ **c.** The spinal nerve forms at the intervertebral foramen.
- ☐ **d.** The anterior primary ramus carries purely motor fibres.
- ☐ **e.** The posterior primary rami never contribute to any innervation of a limb.

7.23 Which statement regarding the sympathetic nervous system is *incorrect*?

- ☐ **a.** There is no sympathetic outflow from the cranial region.
- ☐ **b.** Efferent fibres run in the anterior nerve roots.
- ☐ **c.** Preganglionic fibres run in the grey rami communicantes.
- ☐ **d.** The sympathetic trunk extends from the base of the skull to the coccyx.
- ☐ **e.** Every sympathetic trunk ganglion gives a visceral branch.

7.24 Which statement about the parasympathetic nervous system is *incorrect*?

- ☐ **a.** There is a cranial and a sacral component.
- ☐ **b.** There is no parasympathetic innervation of the limbs.
- ☐ **c.** Preganglionic fibres synapse at or very close to their target.
- ☐ **d.** There are three named parasympathetic ganglia in the cranium.
- ☐ **e.** Outflow from S2–S4 conveys parasympathetic fibres to the pelvic organs.

7.25 Which statement about the tracts of the spinal cord is accurate?

- ☐ **a.** The majority of motor fibres descend in the anterior part of the cord.
- ☐ **b.** The gracile tract lies lateral to the cuneate tract.
- ☐ **c.** The spinothalamic tract carries first order sensory neurones.
- ☐ **d.** The spinothalamic tract subserves pain sensation.
- ☐ **e.** The dorsal columns carry decussated fibres.

7.26 Regarding curvatures of the vertebral column, which statement is *not* correct?

- ☐ **a.** The thoracic and sacrococcygeal curvatures are secondary curvatures.
- ☐ **b.** The cervical curvature becomes prominent before the lumbar curvature.
- ☐ **c.** A kyphosis is characterised by a pathological increase of the thoracic curvature.
- ☐ **d.** A lordosis is characterised by an abnormal increase in lumbar curvature.
- ☐ **e.** A scoliosis is characterised by an abnormal lateral curvature of the column.

7.27 Which statement about the atlas and axis is correct?
- [ ] **a.** The atlas and axis both have no vertebral body.
- [ ] **b.** Rotation of the skull occurs at the atlanto-occipital joint.
- [ ] **c.** The odontoid process (dens) of the axis is weight bearing.
- [ ] **d.** The cruciform ligament holds the dens in position.
- [ ] **e.** There is a vertebral disc between the atlas and axis.

7.28 Which statement regarding cervical vertebrae is *incorrect*?
- [ ] **a.** There are seven cervical vertebrae.
- [ ] **b.** They typically have a bifid spine.
- [ ] **c.** They all have a transverse foramen.
- [ ] **d.** The vertebral body is larger than the vertebral foramen.
- [ ] **e.** There are a total of three atypical cervical vertebrae.

7.29 When considering a typical thoracic vertebrae, which of the following is most accurate?
- [ ] **a.** It has a round body.
- [ ] **b.** Costal facets are a typical feature.
- [ ] **c.** It articulates with its named rib and the rib above.
- [ ] **d.** The 1st thoracic vertebra is a good example.
- [ ] **e.** The transverse processes project laterally and anteriorly.

7.30 Which of the following best describes a feature of a typical lumbar vertebrae?
- [ ] **a.** They have heart-shaped bodies.
- [ ] **b.** The transverse processes get progressively longer to L5.
- [ ] **c.** The spinous processes angle inferiorly.
- [ ] **d.** The vertebral foramen is smaller than that of the cervical vertebrae.
- [ ] **e.** Lumbarisation occurs when the 5th lumbar vertebrae becomes fused to the sacrum.

7.31 Which statement about the sacrum is *incorrect*?

☐ **a.** The sacrum is formed by the fusion of 5 sacral vertebrae.

☐ **b.** The sacral promontory refers to the anterior edge of the 1st sacral vertebra.

☐ **c.** On both surfaces there are five pairs of sacral foramina.

☐ **d.** The sacral canal contains the dural sheath as inferiorly as S2.

☐ **e.** The sacral hiatus is easily located.

7.32 Regarding the joints and ligaments of the vertebral column:

☐ **a.** There are intervertebral discs between all vertebrae above the sacrum.

☐ **b.** Prolapse of the discs tends to occur anteriorly.

☐ **c.** The anterior longitudinal ligament runs from the sacrum to the occipital bone.

☐ **d.** The posterior longitudinal ligament attaches along the spinous processes.

☐ **e.** The ligamentum flavum links adjacent vertebral spines.

ANSWERS

7.1

c. The grey matter represents the cell bodies of the cerebral cortex and covers all surfaces of the hemispheres. Grey matter is found internally in regions such as the thalamus and basal ganglia.

Explanations

a. The cerebral hemispheres occupy the majority of the cranial cavity, but do not occupy any of the posterior cranial fossa. The posterior fossa is the area beneath the tentorium cerebelli and is occupied by the cerebellum and brainstem.

b. The falx cerebri is a fold of dura mater, which separates the two hemispheres. The hemispheres are joined below the falx cerebri by the corpus callosum.

d. The central sulcus separates the frontal lobe from the parietal lobe. The pre- and postcentral gyri are positioned anterior and posterior to the sulcus; they contain the primary motor and somatosensory cortices, respectively.

e. The lateral sulcus separates the temporal lobe from the frontal lobe anteriorly and parietal lobe posteriorly. The occipital lobe lies behind and below the parieto-occipital sulcus.

7.2

a. The primary motor cortex is located in the precentral gyrus of the frontal lobe and is concerned with voluntary movement. Lesions of the cortex produce contralateral weakness.

Explanations

b. The primary somatosensory cortex lies in the postcentral gyrus of the parietal lobe. Lesions of the cortex will produce a contralateral sensory deficit.

c. The primary auditory cortex is responsible for auditory perception and is located in the superior temporal gyrus in the temporal lobe.

d. The primary visual cortex is located in the occipital lobe above and below the calcarine sulcus. Lesions will affect vision on the contralateral field of vision, resulting clinically in a contralateral homonymous hemianopia.

e. Broca's area is located in the inferolateral part of the frontal lobe. Lesions affecting Broca's area result in an expressive dysphasia.

7.3

a. The cerebellum is comprised of two hemispheres joined in the midline by the vermis. It occupies the posterior cranial fossa with the brainstem, and its essential function is the coordination of movement.

Explanations

b. Each cerebellar hemisphere is attached by three pedicles to the three parts of the brainstem. The superior peduncle enters the midbrain, the middle peduncle enters the pons and the inferior peduncle connects the medulla.

c. The small anterior lobe, located on the superior surface, is separated from the larger posterior lobe by the primary fissure. The horizontal fissure, which indents the posterior border, is of no functional significance.

d. The tonsil of the cerebellum is located on the inferior surface of the posterior lobe. It may be displaced inferiorly and herniate through the foramen magnum with a rise in intracranial pressure.

e. The blood supply for the cerebellum is derived from the posterior inferior cerebellar branches of the vertebral artery and the anterior inferior cerebellar and superior cerebellar branches of the basilar artery.

7.4

c. The 4th ventricle sits anterior to the cerebellum and communicates directly with the subarachnoid space via the median foramen of Magendie and two lateral foramina of Luschka.

Explanations

a. CSF is predominantly produced by the choroid plexi of the lateral, 3rd and 4th ventricle.

b. CSF passes from the two lateral ventricles into the 3rd ventricle via the interventricular foramina. The CSF then drains from the 3rd ventricle into the 4th via the cerebral aqueduct of Sylvius, situated in the midbrain.

d. The total volume of CSF is approximately 150 ml, with about 30–40 ml within the ventricular system. This CSF is being continually reabsorbed, with the total daily production in the region of 500 ml. Obstruction to the ventricular system or reabsorption of CSF therefore quickly results in hydrocephalus.

e. Arachnoid granulations are most numerous in the superior sagittal sinus. They represent herniations of arachnoid mater through the dura mater and allow absorption of CSF into the venous system.

7.5

e. The dura continues to terminate distally at the level of the 2nd sacral vertebra. The pia mater tapers to form the filum terminale at the inferior end of the cord, which then continues distally to pierce the dura and insert onto the coccyx.

Explanations

a. The dura mater is the fibrous outermost layer of the meninges. Within the cranium it has an outer endosteal layer and an inner meningeal layer. At the foramen magnum only the inner layer continues inferiorly to cover the cord.

b. The major venous sinuses lie between the two layers of dura mater. The superior cerebral vein crosses the subdural space to empty into the superior sagittal sinus and may result in a subdural haemorrhage if damaged.

c. The middle meningeal artery runs between the dural layers, but bulges through the outer layer and grooves the cranium. Damage to this vessel, for example, in fractures of the pterion; result in an extradural haemorrhage.

d. The pia mater, which intimately lines the brain and spinal cord, is thickened either side of the cord between nerve roots. These denticulate ligaments adhere to the dura and help tether the spinal cord within the sheath.

7.6

c. The pituitary gland sits in the pituitary fossa of the sphenoid bone. Below this is the body of the sphenoid containing the sphenoidal air sinuses. This allows the resection of pituitary tumours via a trans-sphenoidal approach.

Explanations

a. The anterior lobe of the pituitary accounts for about 75% of the total gland. It is connected to the smaller posterior lobe by the narrow pars intermedia.

b. The posterior lobe develops as a cerebral diverticulum and consists of nerve fibres, whose bodies are located in the hypothalamus. The pituitary stalk passes through the diaphragma sellae, a fold of dura mater, and conveys these fibres from the hypothalamus inferiorly.

d. Only the posterior lobe is a cerebral diverticulum. The anterior lobe develops from an ectodermal saccule, Rathke's pouch, in the roof of the primitive buccal cavity. Craniopharyngiomas grow from the pouch remnants.

e. The pituitary gland is related superiorly to the optic chiasm. Enlargement of the pituitary will result in compression of the optic chiasm, leading to presentation with a bitemporal hemianopia.

7.7

c. The term "anterior circulation" refers to the internal carotids and their branches. The term "posterior circulation" refers to the vertebrobasilar system and its branches.

Explanations

a. The circle is formed by the terminal branches of the internal carotid and basilar arteries. The vertebral arteries unite anterior to the upper medulla to become the basilar artery.

b. The ophthalmic artery is a direct branch of the internal carotid artery. The anterior, middle and posterior cerebral arteries form the circle of Willis. They are connected by the anterior and posterior communicating arteries.

d. The posterior cerebral artery largely supplies the occipital lobe. The middle cerebral supplies most of the lateral surface of the cerebral hemispheres.

e. The cerebellar arteries arising from the basilar and vertebral arteries supply the cerebellum.

7.8

d. The arachnoid granulations project into the superior sagittal sinus. This is one of the mechanisms through which CSF drains into the venous circulation.

Explanations

a. The superior sagittal sinus usually drains into the right transverse sinus. The straight sinus usually drains into the left transverse sinus.

b. The great cerebral vein (of Galen) drains along with the inferior sagittal sinus into the straight sinus.

c. The superior petrosal sinuses drain the cavernous sinus into the sigmoid sinuses. The inferior petrosal sinus drains blood from the cavernous sinus into the internal jugular vein.

e. The superior cerebral veins drain the superior part of the brain and empty into the superior sagittal sinus. The superficial middle cerebral veins drain into the cavernous sinus from above.

7.9

b. This presents a potential route of infection between the subarachnoid space and the nasal cavity.

Explanations

a. They pass through the cribriform plate of the ethmoid bone.

c. They run on the inferior surface of the frontal lobes.

d. Bilateral anosmia is commonly associated with anterior cranial fossa fractures due to severance of the olfactory nerves. Unilateral anosmia is more commonly associated with frontal lobe tumours.

e. The primary olfactory cortex is found in the anterior part, or uncus, of the temporal lone. Temporal lobe epilepsy can therefore cause olfactory hallucinations (so called "uncinate" type fits).

7.10

a. The optic nerve is formed by axons of the ganglion cells of the superficial layer of the retina. These fibres converge on the optic disc to form the optic nerve.

Explanations

b. The medial fibres of the optic nerve cross in the optic chiasm. These fibres subserve vision from the temporal visual field. For this reason a lesion compressing the optic chiasm (e.g. a pituitary tumour) causes a bitemporal hemianopia.

c. The majority of the fibres in the optic tract end in the lateral geniculate body in the thalamus. A small number of fibres do pass to the pretectal area and the superior colliculus of the brainstem. These fibres mediate reflex responses to visual stimuli.

d. The optic radiation consists of fibres carrying impulses from the lateral geniculate body to the occipital cortex.

e. The lower part of the retina is represented in the occipital cortex below the calcarine fissure. The upper part of the retina is represented above it.

7.11

e. The parasympathetic fibres are conveyed via the branch to inferior oblique. After synapsing in the ciliary ganglion they supply the ciliary muscles and constrictor pupillae via the short ciliary nerves.

Explanations

a. The oculomotor nerve has two nuclei: the somatic efferent nucleus (supplying superior, inferior and medial rectus, the inferior oblique and the levator palpebrae superioris muscles) and the Edinger–Westphal nucleus (parasympathetic), which lie in the midbrain at the level of the superior colliculus.

b. After emerging from the midbrain the nerve passes between the posterior cerebral and superior cerebellar arteries, and runs forward on the lateral side of the posterior communicating artery. These close relations account for the third nerve palsy that can accompany an aneurysm of any of these vessels.

c. After running through the lateral wall of the cavernous sinus, the nerve divides into a small superior and large inferior division before entering the superior orbital fissure.

d. This is due to unopposed action of dilator pupillae which is supplied by the sympathetic nervous system.

7.12
e. The trochlear nerve enters the orbit through the superior orbital fissure. It runs lateral to the tendinous ring with the lacrimal nerve, frontal nerve and the superior ophthalmic vein.

Explanations
a. The nucleus lies in the midbrain at the level of the inferior colliculus, below that of the oculomotor nerve, which is found at the level of the superior colliculus.
b. The nerve fibres decussate in the superior medullary vellum, having passed around the cerebral aqueduct.
c. The trochlear is the only cranial nerve to emerge on the posterior aspect of the brainstem. It therefore has a long intracranial course and is vulnerable to damage.
d. It runs in the wall of the cavernous sinus along with the oculomotor, ophthalmic and maxillary nerves. The abducent nerve runs through the body of the cavernous sinus along with the internal carotid artery.

7.13
a. The submandibular ganglion is connected to the mandibular nerve.

Explanations
b. The maxillary nerve supplies the upper teeth via its superior alveolar (dental) branches.
c. The greater palatine nerve is a branch from the pterygopalatine ganglion and supplies all the hard palate.
d. The lesser palatine nerve is a branch from the pterygopalatine ganglion and supplies the soft palate.
e. The terminal branch is the infra-orbital nerve. This passes through the inferior orbital fissure to reach the face.

7.14
c. Taste for the anterior 2/3 of the tongue is conveyed by the lingual nerve by fibres which join it from the chorda tympani (VII).

Explanations

a. On exiting the skull through the foramen ovale the mandibular nerve gives a separate branch to supply the medial pterygoid muscle, before dividing into anterior and posterior divisions. The anterior division supplies the other three muscles of mastication (lateral pterygoid, masseter and temporalis) and terminates as the buccal nerve.

b. The auriculo-temporal branch divides briefly to encircle the middle meningeal artery.

d. The posterior belly of digastric is innervated by a branch of the facial nerve. The inferior alveolar branch of the posterior division of the mandibular nerve gives off the nerve to mylohyoid just prior to entering the mandible. This branch supplies the named muscle, and the anterior belly of digastric.

e. The inferior alveolar branch exits the mandible through the mental foramen as the mental nerve, supplying the skin of the chin and lower lip. It enters the mandible via the inferior alveolar or mandibular foramen.

7.15

c. It passes through the tendinous ring with the superior and inferior divisions of the oculomotor nerve and the nasociliary nerve.

Explanations

a. The abducent nerve passes through the body of the cavernous sinus, where it lies lateral to the internal carotid artery.

b. The abducent nerve innervates the lateral rectus. This muscle abducts the eye, which gives the nerve its name.

d. The abducent nerve emerges at the junction between the pons and the medulla.

e. Diplopia occurs on looking to the ipsilateral side as paralysis of the lateral rectus prevents the eye turning outwards.

7.16

b. The statement is correct.

Explanations

a. The chorda tympani nerve conveys parasympathetic fibres for the submandibular and sublingual glands, which synapse in the submandibular ganglion. The lingual nerve then conveys these fibres to the submandibular and sublingual glands.

c. It gives off five main branches within the substance of the parotid gland to supply the muscles of facial expression (temporal, zygomatic, buccal, marginal mandibular and cervical). However, before entering the parotid it gives off two branches to supply the muscles of the auricle, stylohyoid and the posterior belly of digastric.

d. It lies superficial to both the retromandibular vein and external carotid artery within the substance of the parotid, and is therefore extremely vulnerable during parotidectomy.

e. Supranuclear palsies affect the contralateral facial muscles, with sparing of the muscles above the palpebral fissure, since the portion of the facial nucleus supplying these muscles receives fibres from both cerebral hemispheres.

7.17

b. The vestibulocochlear nerve enters the medulla at the cerebellopontine angle with the facial nerve. For this reason an acoustic neuroma can compress the facial nerve causing ipsilateral facial weakness.

Explanations

a. The vestibulocochlear nerve is made up of two groups of fibres. The cochlear fibres arise from the spiral ganglion cells of the cochlea and subserve hearing. The vestibular fibres subserve balance.

c. The auditory radiation passes between these two structures. Temporal lobe tumours or temporal lobe epilepsy can therefore cause auditory hallucinations.

d. For this reason unilateral lesions of the auditory pathway above the cochlear nerve do not cause any deafness.

e. The vestibular nerve terminates in the vestibular nucleus, efferent fibres from this nucleus pass to the cerebellum. This connection is important in maintaining balance.

7.18

d. The glossopharyngeal nerve is one of the structures separating the internal and external carotid arteries. The others are the pharyngeal branch of the vagus, the stylopharyngeus muscle and the styloid process of the temporal bone.

Explanations

a. The glossopharyngeal nerve supplies preganglionic fibres to the otic ganglion via its lesser petrosal branch. Postganglionic fibres are conveyed by the auriculotemporal nerve to the parotid gland.

b. The glossopharyngeal nerve innervates stylopharyngeus.

c. It supplies the carotid body chemoreceptors and carotid sinus baroreceptors.

e. The lingual branch of the glossopharyngeal nerve supplies common sensation and taste to the posterior 1/3 of the tongue.

7.19

a. The vagus nerve is deep to the carotid artery and internal jugular vein in the carotid sheath.

Explanations

b. The vagus nerve passes in front of the subclavian artery on both sides.

c. The vagus has an auricular branch which contributes to the sensory supply of the external surface of the tympanic membrane.

d. The right recurrent laryngeal nerve is given off as the right vagus crosses the subclavian artery and hooks around this vessel. The left recurrent laryngeal nerve is given off in the superior mediastinum and hooks under the arch of the aorta, around the ligamentum arteriosum.

e. The recurrent laryngeal nerve supplies all the intrinsic muscles of the larynx except the cricothyroid, which is supplied by the external branch of the superior laryngeal nerve. Both of these nerves are branches of the vagus.

7.20

c. These fibres do not join the vagus but pass deep to the posterior belly of digastric and the styloid process to enter the sternocleidomastoid.

Explanations

a. The spinal root enters the skull through the foramen magnum, it joins the cranial root just before the accessory nerve leaves the skull through the jugular foramen.

b. The cranial root is distributed via the vagus nerve and carries fibres which are thought to be motor to the muscles in the pharynx, larynx and palate.

d. The cranial root joins the vagus nerve. The spinal root pierces, and innervates, sternocleidomastoid.

e. The spinal root passes across the posterior triangle of the neck, having left the sternocleidomastoid, and supplies trapezius. It is vulnerable to surgical damage in this region.

7.21

d. The anterior and posterior nerve roots emerge from the cord and pass to the intervertebral foramina, where they unite to form the segmental spinal nerve. The length of these roots increases inferiorly to reflect the difference between the length of spinal cord and that of the vertebral column.

Explanations

a. The spinal cord is the continuation of the medulla oblongata and descends to taper into the conus medullaris at the junction between the 1st and 2nd lumbar vertebrae in adults. This is at approximately level L3 in the newborn.

b. The spinal cord is largely supplied by the single anterior and paired posterior spinal arteries. They receive important reinforcement by radicular branches of various other arteries as the cord descends. The radicular branches may be damaged during operations on the vertebral column or adjacent structures, severely compromising the blood supply of the cord.

c. There are two important symmetrical enlargements which occupy the segments of the limb plexi: the cervical and lumbosacral plexi. The enlargements are due to a large increase in motor cells in the anterior horn cells of grey matter at these points.

e. The spinal roots unite to form the spinal nerve, and exit through the intervertebral foramina. The vertebral foramen contains the cord itself.

7.22

d. Both the anterior and posterior rami carry both motor and sensory fibres.

Explanations

a. There are 8 cervical, 12 thoracic, 5 lumbar, 5 sacral and 1 coccygeal pairs. Rootlets emerging from the cord contribute to anterior and posterior roots, which combine to form the spinal nerve.

b. The posterior root contains sensory afferent fibres and the anterior root contains motor efferent fibres. There is a ganglion on the posterior root, known as the posterior root ganglion, which contains the cell bodies of the afferent sensory nerves.

c. The two roots unite at the intervertebral foramen. They then divided into anterior and posterior primary rami, which carry a mixture of motor and sensory fibres.

e. The posterior rami innervate the intrinsic muscles of the back and neck, along with the overlying skin in the paravertebral gutter. The anterior rami innervate all of the other muscles of the trunk and limbs, and the remaining skin (except that innervated by the trigeminal nerve on the face).

7.23

c. Preganglionic fibres are myelinated and therefore appear white. They leave the anterior primary ramus to run in the white rami communicantes to enter the sympathetic trunk. Postganglionic fibres are unmyelinated and appear grey running in the grey rami communicantes to rejoin the relevant spinal nerve.

Explanations

a. The sympathetic preganglionic cell bodies are located in the lateral horn cells of all the thoracic and upper two lumbar cord segments.

b. The efferent preganglionic fibres run in the anterior nerve root to enter the spinal nerve and its anterior primary ramus.

d. There is no sympathetic outflow from the cervical or lower lumbar and sacral parts of the cord. The preganglionic fibres for these regions must travel in the sympathetic trunk to ganglia at the appropriate level.

e. In the cervical and upper thoracic regions, cardiac branches descend to the cardiac plexus. From the lower ganglia visceral branches coalesce to form splanchnic nerves, which descend to the coeliac, superior and inferior hypogastric plexi.

7.24

d. The cranial parasympathetic outflow is conveyed by cranial nerves III, XII, IX and X. Parasympathetic fibres from the first three synapse in four ganglia to send postganglionic fibres to innervate the eye and salivary and lacrimal ducts. These are the ciliary, pterygopalatine, submandibular and otic ganglia.

Explanations

a. The parasympathetic component of the autonomic nervous system has a cranial and sacral component.

b. While all parts of the body receive sympathetic innervation, parasympathetic supply is purely visceral. No parasympathetic fibres are distributed to the limbs or trunk.

c. Unlike the sympathetic system, where postganglionic fibres often have a long, convoluted path to their target, parasympathetic preganglionic fibres synapse at ganglia at or very close to their target organ.

e. The sacral preganglionic fibres arise from the sacral segments S2–S4 in fibres known as the pelvic splanchnic nerves. These fibres are distributed via the sympathetic plexi to innervate the pelvic viscera.

7.25

d. The spinothalamic tract subserves pain, temperature and crude touch.

Explanations

a. The majority of motor fibres descend in pyramidal tract in the lateral part of the cord, having decussated in the medulla. A minority, approximately 15%, descend without decussating in the anterior part of the cord.

b. The gracile tract lies medial to the cuneate tract. The gracile and cuneate tracts form the dorsal columns. They carry fibres subserving fine touch, vibration and proprioception.

c. The fibres in the spinothalamic tract ascend two or three segments and synapse with a second order neurone. This neurone then decussates and either ascends to synapse in the thalamus or in the brainstem. Fibres from the thalamus are relayed to the sensory cortex by a third order neurone.

e. The fibres in the dorsal columns are undecussated. They decussate in the medulla where a second order neurone carries fibres to the thalamus. A third order neurone then carries fibres from the thalamus to the cerebral cortex.

7.26

a. They are primary curvatures which develop as a result of the normal foetal position within the uterus.

Explanations

b. After birth secondary extension of the column produces secondary curvatures, which are convex anteriorly. The cervical curvature becomes prominent as the infant begins to hold its head erect, and the lumbar curvature emerges as the infant assumes an upright posture as it learns to walk.

c. A kyphosis represents an abnormal increase in the thoracic curvature. It occurs due to erosion of the anterior portion of one or more vertebrae, with progressive erosion and collapse leading to a loss of height.

d. Lordosis is characterised by an anterior rotation of the pelvis causing an increase in lumbar curvature. This is commonly seen in the later stages of pregnancy or in the obese patient, where the extra weight lies anterior to the normal line of gravity.

e. A scoliosis is the result of an abnormal lateral curvature of the vertebral column. This is accompanied by rotation of the vertebrae.

7.27

d. The transverse ligament runs between the inner aspects of the lateral masses of the atlas, grooving the posterior aspect of the dens. The weaker longitudinal ligament runs from the posterior body of the axis to the basiocciput and together they form the cruciform ligament. Rupture of the ligament allows posterior dislocation of the dens with fatal consequences.

Explanations

a. The atlas has no vertebral body. The axis has the odontoid process (dens) arising from the superior aspect of its body. The dens represents the detached remnant of the body of the atlas.

b. Rotation of the skull occurs at the synovial atlanto-axial joint around the dens. Head nodding occurs at the synovial atlanto-occipital joint.

c. The odontoid process is entirely non-weight bearing. The weight of the skull is transmitted via the lateral masses of the atlas, to the superior articular facets of the axis, either side of the dens.

e. The first vertebral disc is between the axis and C3.

7.28

d. The body of a typical cervical vertebra is described as kidney shaped and is the same size or smaller than its vertebral foramen. The foramen is ample in order to transmit the still substantial spinal cord.

Explanations

a. There are seven cervical vertebrae, but eight cervical spinal nerves. The 1st cervical nerve exits above C1, but the 1st thoracic nerve exits below T1. The 8th cervical nerve, therefore, exits between C7 and T1.

b. A feature of the typical cervical vertebrae is the presence of a small, bifid spinous process. The exceptions are the C1 (atlas) and C7 (vertebra prominens) vertebrae, which have non-bifid spines.

c. All cervical vertebrae have a transverse foramen perforating their transverse process. The vertebral artery runs in the neck through the transverse foramina of C1–C6 with its accompanying vein. However, only the vein continues through that of C7, and hence this foramen is often much smaller or even absent.

e. There are three atypical vertebrae: the atlas (C1), the axis (C2) and the vertebra prominens (C7), so called because it has a long and easily palpable spine.

7.29

b. On each side of a typical thoracic vertebra there are a pair of semicircular demifacets. The upper is found at the junction of the pedicle and the body, and articulates with the head of the corresponding rib. The smaller facet is at the lower border of the body and articulates with the head of the rib below.

Explanations

a. Both the anterior and posterior aspects of the body of the thoracic vertebrae are concave anteriorly, thus giving them a heart-shaped appearance. This produces a characteristic circular vertebral foramen between body and lamina.

c. The ribs articulate with the vertebral bodies as described in 7.29b, with the tubercle on the neck of the corresponding rib also articulating with the transverse process of its named vertebrae.

d. The 1st thoracic vertebra is considered atypical. The body is broad and not heart shaped, and the upper costal facet is enlarged and rounded to articulate with the 1st rib (which does not articulate with the body of C7). The 10th, 11th and 12th vertebrae are also considered atypical.

e. The transverse processes project laterally and posteriorly, and expand at their tips to carry the transverse costal facet.

7.30

d. The lumbar vertebral foramina are triangular in shape and while larger than those of the thoracic vertebrae, they are smaller than those of the cervical vertebrae.

Explanations

a. The lumbar vertebral bodies are kidney shaped and increase in breadth from above down. Heart-shaped bodies are a characteristic feature of thoracic vertebrae.

b. The transverse processes project straight laterally and get progressively longer to L4. The atypical 5th lumbar vertebra has short, massive, triangular transverse processes, which are unique in joining to the vertebral body itself.

c. The spinous processes a short and project straight posteriorly.

e. Sacralisation describes the condition where the 5th lumbar vertebra becomes fused to the sacrum. Lumbarisation is the rarer condition describing the presence of a distinct, separated, 1st sacral vertebra.

7.31

c. There are four pairs of sacral foramina on both surfaces to allow for the exit of the first four anterior and posterior sacral rami, respectively. The 5th sacral nerve is transmitted through the sacral hiatus, at the inferior end of the sacral canal.

Explanations

a. The sacrum is described as wedge or triangle shaped and is formed by the fusion of five sacral vertebrae. It functions to provide stability and strength to the pelvis.

b. The sacral promontory is the protruding anterior edge of the 1st sacral vertebrae and is a readily palpable landmark during laparotomy.

d. The sacral canal is the continuation of the inferior end of the vertebral canal. The dural sheath terminates at the level of the 2nd sacral vertebra and the remaining canal is filled with extradural fat.

e. The sacral hiatus leads into the sacral canal. It can be easily located by palpating the sacral cornua either side of the hiatus above the natal cleft. An injection of anaesthetic into the hiatus will target the lower spinal roots as they emerge from the end of the dural sheath and may be of use during difficult or traumatic childbirth.

7.32

c. This strong fibrous band extends from the anterior surface of the sacrum to the occipital bone anterior to the foramen magnum. It prevents hyperextension and maintains the stability of the vertebral column.

Explanations

a. There is no articular disc between the 1st and 2nd cervical vertebrae. The discs are extremely important structures, not only accounting for approximately 1/4 of the length of the spine, but also contributing the secondary curvatures.

b. The discs consist of a peripheral annulus fibrosus composed of fibrocartilage, which surrounds a gelatinous nucleus pulposus. The annulus fibrosus is thinnest posteriorly and may rupture as a result of degenerative or traumatic changes, permitting herniation of the nucleus pulposus posteriorly. The prolapsed disc may impinge on the nerve root emerging at that level.

d. The supraspinous ligament connects the spinous processes. The posterior longitudinal ligament runs along the posterior aspect of the vertebral bodies, within the vertebral canal. It prevents hyperflexion of the column and protrusion of the discs.

e. The ligament connects adjacent vertebral laminae. The ligamentum flavum is unique in the body as it is a yellow rather than a white ligament. This is because it contains elastin. This elastic ligament allows flexion of the spine while providing support.